MEDICAL STUDENT LOANS

A COMPREHENSIVE GUIDE

BEN WHITE, MD

Medical Student Loans: A Comprehensive Guide
Ben White, M.D.
Copyright © 2017 by Benjamin White, M.D.
Published by BWMD LLC
Last revision: November 2019
Cover Photo Credit: Pictures of Money
(CheapFullCoverageAutoInsurance.com [yes, really])

Disclaimer: Disclaimers are worthless. And yet, I feel obligated to inform you that the material in this book is the work of a fallible individual and is intended for informational purposes only. Nothing contained herein should be construed for financial, legal, or even medical advice. I am not a "Certified Student Loan Professional" and have no interest in being one. Even though there appear to be multiple recommendations throughout the book including lots of numbers and basic arithmetic, none of that is *really* financial advice. I promise.

Transparency Disclosure: I maintain a lightly-monetized for-profit personal website, and I periodically make a small amount of money from referrals to student loan refinancing companies.

Visit: www.benwhite.com

Correspondence: ben@benwhite.com

For Noah,
I wasn't living a full life until you were in it.

TABLE OF CONTENTS

INTRODUCTION

In 2016, the average graduating medical student owed $190,000 in student loans, and 40% of graduates planned on loan forgiveness. And when the AAMC says $190,000, they mean the average amount *borrowed* for school is $190,000, not the amount the average student graduates with (which is already closer to $215,000 due to interest accruing during school). Student loan debt is a big issue and a big industry with no signs of slowing down. That original "$190,000," if paid over a standard 10-year repayment, would end up costing $2400 a month for a total $291k. Given that most residents can't afford the standard repayment, spending that little on interest would be a dream for many borrowers, especially since many students are far away from the average reported on the AAMC's little survey. Dealing with medical student loans is a long process with a lot of money at stake.

It's not so much that managing student loans is particularly complicated. It's not acid/base physiology, and there are only a few options available. The issue is that the correct choice depends on your personal circumstances, including how much you owe, to whom, how much you earn, how long your training is, your marital status, and what kind of job you plan on having. There is no substitute for sitting down and running some numbers yourself, testing some assumptions and possibilities, and reevaluating your plan whenever your circumstances change.

So, you don't need this book. In fact, no one needs any book on student loans. What you really need is to periodically sit down and think about how to handle your debt and be prepared to Google. But I wrote this book to save the Googling and get all the facts, options, and considerations in one hopefully easy-to-read package. Misinformation runs rampant. Just like how you want patients who are invested in their wellbeing, you should be an active participant in your financial health.

Doctors are in a unique position: they incur a very large load of debt in exchange for a near guarantee of a solid but generally not ridiculous long-term income. In between, they have several years of comparatively paltry earnings during residency. The average resident will either forbear (not pay) their loans during residency and then begin making payments as an attending or pick an income-driven repayment plan at the outset and stay on it indefinitely. Both of these options will work in the sense that you will eventually pay off your debt, but a few hours of reading now and some intermittent consideration later can both save you money in the long run and give you the mental satisfaction of knowing you're taking care of your reverse nest egg as best you can.

But let's be real: no one has a monopoly on this information (the core of which is provided for free by the government). What you probably can't do yet is find any one place to get a complete up-to-date one-stop-shop for how to handle your student loan debt in a handy organized format with multiple examples to illustrate your options. In short, this short book was a big effort.

Some final thoughts to keep in mind before we dive in:

- Even though this book appears to be full of financial and even tax advice, it isn't. That's a clever optical and semantic illusion. Nothing within this book should be construed as or serve as a replacement for "real" advice from a "professional," which honestly you probably don't need and shouldn't buy, because ick.

- As a rule, every illustration in this book and every best practice when it comes to managing your finances changes/depends on several factors, including your marital status and how much your spouse earns if they work. Everything from your tax deductions to your calculated loan payments will all depend on family size, marital status, and gross income.

- It isn't possible to give illustrative examples that will apply to every reader. I frequently refer to an average loan of $200,000 with a fixed interest rate of 6.0%. This is because it's a nice round number near the current average student loan debt, and 6.0% is near what a new graduate with that much debt would have as an average rate. We're trying to keep things simple. You can adjust my numbers and illustrations a bit in your head, but it is seriously in your best interest to sit down at some point and really run your numbers for yourself. No illustration is a substitute for that. We'll talk about how to do that later.

- Some of the if-this then-thats in this book are repetitive, and important facets are repeated every time they're relevant. I'm okay with that. I'd rather be a little boring than lose anyone when it counts.

Some parts are extremely basic.

Other portions are very granular.

My hope is that whatever your background that some part of this book will help you consider how to handle the big investment you've made in yourself.

CONTEXT

Not too long ago, my wife and I were medical students living off our student loans. Now, we're doctors with a toddler and even bigger loans (thanks, negative amortization). This book, which grew out of over eight years of writing about student loans online, exists because for some unknown reason the Internet is full of tripe when it comes to student loan management, and most (but not all) of the good stuff isn't tailored to doctors and their unique situation of very high debt, temporarily low income, then relatively high income.

There is a smattering of useful government resources with most of the core information you need spread across multiple pages on multiple sites but frequently short on details, a plethora of terrible forum posts and comment threads where the blind lead the blind, and a bunch of websites shamelessly trying to make money off you, including a bunch of companies trying to profit by helping you "qualify" for the federal government programs that you're always entitled to for free. Others are student loan consultants who want you to pay them to help you figure out what you can do for yourself. And finally, there are the sites that are theoretically informational but are also heavily monetized by ads or private refinancing arrangements and filled with frequent and often reader-hostile clickbait posts about the "top 10 mistakes" borrowers make or the "one weird trick" to blasting your student loans. This isn't to say there's anything wrong with private refinancing, because there isn't. It's the right move for some people, and we'll discuss it at length in this book, but there's a difference between discussing it (or even promoting it) and making it a business model.

And speaking of financial affiliations, my pot-calling-the-kettle disclosure: my website also sometimes earns money from relationships with private refinance companies. To be generally helpful, I've always set up these partnerships to split any referral bonuses I would receive in favor of the readers who refinance through them. I don't believe these arrangements inform my writing, but we'll discuss this again in the private refinance chapter, because transparency is important. This is something I've been able to arrange because of the readership of my site. It's not a significant part of my livelihood, which comes from practicing medicine like you, but it is an obvious conflict of interest.

A STUDENT LOAN STORY

Let's begin with the story of Ben (any resemblance to any person either living or dead is purely coincidental), a pretty "average" doctor. Between scholarships and parental help, he finished his undergraduate studies debt free.

He borrowed around $40,000 a year at 6.8% to pay for tuition and living expenses for medical school. Because those loans were unsubsidized, that $160,000 turned into $187,000 by the time graduation rolled around.

After graduation, he had a six-month grace period during intern year. That was nice because he had to move across the country and get settled. By then, he owed $192,000 total ($160,000 principal and $32,000 in interest). At the end of that period, the $32,000 in interest capitalized and became part of the principal, meaning that the loan was going to grow a bit faster from this point on.

Because the hours were rough and he was tired of living like a student, he decided to live in a pretty nice apartment near the hospital. He also felt like he needed a newer car because his ancient one was an unreliable clunker without AC and no backup camera. He did the math and realized he wouldn't be able to make payments, so he opted for forbearance throughout residency.

Three years later, he graduated and decided to become a hospitalist. The forbearance period ended—triggering another round of interest capitalization—and his new capitalized loan balance was $231,000.

He decided to be proactive at this point and opt for the standard repayment to pay down his loans in what he considered a timely ten-year fashion. He paid $2,700 a month for 120 months for a total of $319,000, and he was finally student-loan debt-free. That was another $88,000 in interest over the ten years of repayment.

Ultimately, he paid twice what he initially borrowed. That four-dollar Starbucks latte he bought as an MS1 actually cost him eight bucks.

This story illustrates one option, but not a particularly good one. Now that I have your attention, we're going to break down all of the terms and all of your options over the course of this short book.

PROFESSIONAL ADVICE

After you read that little story, you may be wondering with whom you should talk about your loans.

You may have friends from high school or college who are financial advisors who would love to lend you a hand. But even most well-meaning financial folks are not fully versed in the nuances of student loans, and sadly many more financial folks aren't particularly well-meaning. Many financial professionals are more salesman than advisor, so before you pay anyone for anything, you need to be certain how they make their money. If they're trying to sell you insurance or manage your investment accounts, be wary some serious conflicts of interest. Likewise, many student loan "professionals" have negotiated arrangements with student loan companies and get paid commissions on refinanced loans (another COI). You'll generally be safer with a "fee-only" (not just "fee-based") financial advisor, to whom you pay either a flat fee or hourly rate. You also only want one who will act as a "fiduciary," which means they're bound to act in your best interest. Even then, hiring a professional doesn't obviate the need to do your own due diligence.

If someone mentions the words whole life insurance or annuity or wants to actively manage your investments—run, don't walk. First, you don't need someone to manage your assets when you don't have any. And, more importantly, people operating via commission or assets under management who are willing to see you for free or on the cheap in order to establish a relationship with you are not being charitable. Even if you get a free steak dinner, don't ever think you owe anyone anything. This is a marketing expense for them, not a favor to you. Free student loan advice is often worth less than nothing.

The people who on the face of it may seem to be best-suited to help you are those with the new "certified student loan professional" designation. Sounds legit, right? I used to mock the CSLA organization mercilessly in previous versions of this book because its initial addition to the alphabet soup of mostly dubious professional financial accreditations is achieved by taking an online video course and passing a 90-question multiple-choice test. Whew, serious stuff. The website (cslainstitute.org) also used to misspell the RE-PAYE program as "Repay." That said, at least the course content has tightened up to something more meaningful over the years. I *might* trust a financial planner with the CSLP certification more than one without, but you still need to make sure they can walk the walk, and you can't do that if you can't follow the logic.

Any person you pay to help you is going to plug your numbers into a glorified (or actual) Excel spreadsheet. Not only is this something you can do yourself, but any Excel spreadsheet or online calculator is only as useful as its assumptions and inputs, and none meaningfully represents all of your true options.

You have (or will soon have) a doctorate. You may not be a finance buff, but you're smart enough to learn what you need to know. Consider this your first few hours of CME.

In all seriousness, while I believe you can do this yourself, there are definitely people who have complicated situations and would benefit from professional help. You should at least learn enough that you can understand the *why* of what a professional advises. Don't just take things at face value.

GLOSSARY

Before we dive too deep, first let's define some terms. We're doing it at the beginning, just to make sure everyone is on the same page.

Loan - A sum of money you borrow from somebody, typically the federal government or a bank for the majority of student loans.

Interest rate - The rate at which a sum of money grows, usually expressed as a percentage. The higher the rate, the faster it grows. This is great for investments but equally less great for your loans. Most quoted rates are an "annual" percentage. So, a $100,000 loan at 5% APR (annual percentage rate) will accrue $5,000 in interest every year.

Capitalization - Capitalization is when the interest accrued on a loan is added permanently to the "principal" (the loan itself aka the amount that accrues interest). For example, if interest capitalizes annually, then a forbeared/unpaid $100,000 loan with a 5% interest rate accruing $5,000 in unpaid interest would become a $105,000 loan accruing $5,250 the following year. Capitalization is commonly referred to as "compounding" when it works in your favor, such as in an investing account.

The following are events that trigger capitalization:

- End of grace period / beginning of repayment
- End of a period of forbearance or deferment
- Change in repayment plan or consolidation
- Loss of partial financial hardship in IBR or PAYE
- Failure to submit IDR annual income certification on time
- Loan Default

Income-driven repayment (IDR) - An umbrella term for the government's multiple payment plans which tie your monthly payments to your income, which include income-based repayment (IBR), pay as you earn (PAYE), revised pay as you earn (REPAYE), and income-contingent repayment (ICR). The term IBR is sometimes also confusingly used as a stand-in for IDR programs in general, but IBR is actually a specific program under the IDR umbrella.

We'll compare & contrast the IDR programs in detail later, but in brief:

Income-based repayment (IBR) - Monthly payments for most borrowers are calculated to be 15% of discretionary income and are capped to never be greater than the amount you would pay monthly on the standard 10-year plan when you first entered repayment. Loans are forgiven after 25 years of payments.

Pay as you earn (PAYE) - Monthly payments for most borrowers are calculated to be 10% of discretionary income and are capped to never be greater than the amount you would pay monthly on the standard 10-year plan when you first entered repayment. Loans are forgiven after 20 years of payments.

Revised pay as you earn (REPAYE) - The new late 2015 addition to the IDR pantheon. Monthly payments are capped at 10% of your discretionary income like PAYE, but half of the unpaid interest left over after your monthly payment is also forgiven (the unpaid interest subsidy). This sounds better than PAYE, and it often is, but REPAYE also closes some loopholes that make PAYE a better choice for some folks. Undergraduate loans are forgiven after 20 years, but anyone with graduate loans (e.g. you) has to wait 25 years like IBR.

Income-contingent repayment (ICR) – An antiquated nearly irrelevant program. ICR is only really relevant for older students who have older FFEL loans or parents who hold Parent Plus loans. Using ICR to pay off Parent Plus loans that have been consolidated into a Direct Consolidation loan is the only way to get forgiveness for these otherwise inflexible loans (note: the qualifying nonprofit work in this edge case is the *parent's,* not the student's).

Discretionary income - The income amount used to calculate your IDR payments. Discretionary income is calculated as your adjusted gross income (total income before taxes minus deductions) minus 150% of the poverty line. You can find your AGI on your taxes. The poverty line varies by family size (as well as lower 48 vs Hawaii/Alaska). As an example, the 2016 poverty line for an individual was $11,880.

Subsidized loans - Subsidized loans used to be given to graduate students prior to 2012. Now they're reserved for undergrads. Subsidized loans do not accrue interest during school or any other deferment period. Any unpaid interest that accrues during the first three years of IDR after graduation is also completely covered. Subsidized loans are only relevant for recent graduates if they also have loans from college.

Unsubsidized loan - The classic student loan that likely makes up the vast majority of your debt. Interest accrues from the day you take out the money.

Private refinancing - These days the vast majority of student loans are given out by the government as part of the Direct loan program (because they're given "directly" by the government as opposed to given by banks but guaranteed/insured by the government, as used to be the case). Some companies do offer student loans, but these are generally less good than the federal offerings. But some offer private refinancing/consolidation, whereby they pay off your existing student loans in exchange for a loan with a lower interest rate. You can save money, sometimes a lot of money, but you also lose the benefits/flexibility/protections of federal loans including possible forgiveness.

Cosigner - A person who applies for a loan with you in order to help you qualify for a loan you otherwise wouldn't get or help you get a better rate. The cosigner is responsible for the loan just like you and is on the hook if you don't follow through. In some circumstances, companies have programs to remove a cosigner from a loan after a period of on-time payments.

Public service loan forgiveness - A program that (currently) offers unlimited tax-free loan forgiveness to those working at qualifying non-profit organizations after ten years of on-time monthly payments. The very first crop of forgiven loans was eligible in October 2017, but few have made it through the forgiveness gauntlet so far. The future of this program is unknown and frequently discussed.

Deferment is the ideal way to temporarily not pay off your loans. In a deferment (as opposed to forbearance, covered below), no monthly payments are due on your loans and no interest on subsidized loans accrues. In practice, the only deferment you are going to get is the one you have while you are enrolled at least part-time in school. In the past, residents were eligible for an economic hardship deferment. That is no longer the case.

Forbearance is how you can temporarily not make payments on your loans. Most people can only forbear loans for three years, but residents have the use of an unlimited in-training forbearance, so you are never obligated to make payments on your federal student loans while a resident if you feel it's financially unfeasible (though you have to apply annually). The downside is that interest continues to accumulate and then capitalizes at the end of the forbearance period, so your debt balloons more the longer you delay making payments. New attendings who are finally ready to start tackling their student loans are often horrified to see how much their debt has grown after a few years of neglect.

Grace period is the mandatory 6-month period after graduation before you enter repayment. Consolidation and PLUS loans do not have grace periods. Perkins loans have a 9-month grace period.

Repayment is the period during which you make monthly scheduled payments toward your loans after your six-month grace period.

Delinquency is when you miss making a payment, even by one day. Reported to credit agencies. This is one great reason to sign up for autopay.

Default is when you don't handle your delinquency. The entire balance is due *immediately*. At this point, your credit score is shredded for at least seven years *and* the government comes after you to get its money. This includes things like penalties and fees, garnishing your wages, seizing social security, and taking your tax refunds. This should never happen (particularly since you can always forbear as a resident). What many defaulting borrowers fail to realize is that IDR payments can be reduced quickly if income falls; bankruptcies from medical illness aside, the payments are designed to never be totally undoable. If your income is low, your payments are low.

BORROW LESS AND SAVE MORE

This chapter is geared toward current and prospective students, but there's still something in here for everyone.

BORROW LESS TO OWE LESS

This is not really the kind of personal finance book where we spend a lot of time talking about spending less and saving more (though of course, you should). We're also not going to spend much time saying you need to "live like a student" now or "live like a student later." Besides, for a doctor, it's more like, "live like a student now or be forced to remain in the workplace longer than you want, take a job you don't want, or work harder than you want in order to pay your bills and then retire securely."

Your overall net worth—which will almost assuredly be negative for quite some time—will be better if you can live like a student while you're in medical school and borrow accordingly. Trying to keep up a lifestyle with your former classmates who hold real jobs is a losing proposition when you're doing it on credit.

Then, when you're a resident, you'd want to keep living like a student. Ideally. But I'd be lying if I told you that's what I or most reasonable people I know did during residency. However, you should *live like a resident* (and not attending). Don't start or continue spending money you don't have. Not only can you not afford it now, but it's a habit trajectory with no happy ending. You can always spend more.

Hedonic adaptation (getting used to nice things) is a real phenomenon. Improvements to your standard of living bring small increases in happiness followed by rapid habituation. On the other hand, even relatively small lifestyle decreases can bring lasting misery. If you must borrow money to buy something, you can't afford it. For medical school, that was an investment in yourself. For most everything else, it's just you living the false American dream. If you can't pay off your credit card every month, you're spending too much money.

As a student, this means putting serious thought into several things:

1. What kind of school are you going to? Public institution with (relatively) cheap in-state tuition? Private university? Pricey osteopathic school? For-profit Caribbean school?

2. Where is that school located and how much does that city cost to live in? Will you need a car, and if so, how is parking?

A state medical school in an affordable city is going to cost you much less than a private medical school in an expensive city. Most students are so excited to get into medical school that they don't put a thought to the cost when selecting where to go (if they even have options in the first place). Others, wanting to go to the "best" school possible, may also end up picking one with a much bigger sticker price.

You can use a site like StartClass (http://www.startclass.com) to compare tuitions across different institutions.

No matter what sticker price you read, the lag time between the data you use to base cost estimations and what you'll experience is significant. A college student looks at the average graduating debt of $200,000 and may think it's doable. But that was for medical students *who just graduated*, not for students who have yet to start. A student applying in the fall of 2017 will be looking at 2016 data from students who went to school between 2012-16. But they'll be in med school from 2018-2022. That's a six-year lag, and—with inevitable tuition increases—he or she will be paying more. According to the AAMC, average education debt was $190,000 in 2016. It was $157,900 in 2010. That's a 20% increase from what those students might have expected. If the trend continues, we'll be looking at around $230,000 for the class of 2022.

I don't particularly want to get into the politics of whether a big-name school is "worth it" or not. There are reasons it might be. But as a future income & residency-competitiveness calculus, I will simply point out two things: One, medical school is not college. College is both much more variable and much more fun. Two, high-earning physicians in highly competitive fields come from every school. You will or have already done whatever you want, but school choice has a huge impact on how much you'll be investing in your education.

AVOIDING PLUS LOANS

Federal loans for graduate students come in two varieties. The painful Direct Unsubsidized loans and the even more painful Direct PLUS loans, which have higher origination fees and higher interest rates. When you get your student loan information from your school, you'll find out how much they'll give you and in what kind of form. Medical students can borrow up to $40,500 per year up to a $224,000 aggregate total (including undergraduate) in Direct Unsubsidized loans, so if you'll need more than that then you'll be looking at some PLUS loans.

You'll always save money by borrowing less, but this is especially true if you can get by without PLUS loans or by minimizing them.

AVOIDING PRIVATE LOANS

In most cases, private loans are less desirable than even PLUS loans. Rates are frequently higher than government loans. Even worse, these loans lack the flexible payment programs and protections of federal loans and are, of course, ineligible for federal loan forgiveness programs. Seriously reconsider any life plan that requires private loans on top of the usual federal ones.

One potential exception are institutional or organization-based loans, which are often promoted by schools and offered through endowments, foundations, or organizations. These loans often have relatively reasonable rates and are frequently subsidized, but each is unique and must be considered on its own merits. These are especially desirable when extra cash is needed on top of normal borrowing (e.g. fourth year interview travel) but think carefully before utilizing an institutional loan *instead* of a regular direct loan for primary school expenses: the paper terms are likely better, but they will also be ineligible for federal repayment plans and forgiveness. It'll depend on your long-term plans if that matters or not. If you have any, you'll want to wait to refinance them until the end of any subsidized/interest-free period.

THE LOAN FROM THE BANK OF MOM AND DAD

For a variety of reasons, you may be unable or unwilling to borrow money from family. But there's no denying that, if your family has the resources, they would probably offer better terms than a bank. Just saying.

DELAY LOAN DISBURSEMENTS

Typically, student loans are distributed at the beginning of each semester (i.e. twice a year). Obviously, the tuition must come from somewhere, but you don't need to take out your entire six months of living expenses at the very beginning of the term and have it sit accruing interest before you need it. Taking out an extra $20,000 in living expenses at 6% half a year before you need it costs you $600. The more non-tuition money you borrow, the more you can save by not taking it before you need it. This can save thousands over the course of school.

You can request the money from your school when you need it. The turnaround time is usually a few days to a few weeks, and the financial office at your school knows what they can do. Find out from your school how fast they turn around disbursement requests and plan accordingly. While it does require some effort on your part, it's worth it.

CHARGE YOUR LIFE

Gaming the system of credit card interest rates and rewards is the lifeblood of plenty of point hackers and lifestyle bloggers. Using an extreme form of it to pay for medical school was also publicized by the late physician finance blogger Amanda Liu. Because of previous employment, she had access to credit cards with very high charge limits. Her school also allowed her to charge her tuition to a credit card without a fee. She would charge her tuition to a new card with a 0% introductory rate, then at the end of the term, take out the loan to pay off the credit card. This delayed her taking the loan by several months and allowed her to earn thousands of dollars in rewards/perks.

While very clever, her method won't work that way for many people. The first hurdle is that many schools don't allow you to directly charge your tuition to a credit card, and most of the ones that do will pass on a service fee to you, often around 2-4%, wiping away most if not all the benefit.

The workaround to that is a service like Plastiq (www.plastiq.com). Plastiq is an intermediate payment company. They charge your credit card and then issue a check or ACH transfer to pay your bill. In this way, you can use your credit card for any expense even if the recipient doesn't accept credit cards directly. Plastiq charges 2.5% for the privilege, so this doesn't come free, but depending on the bonuses from your card, it can still be worth it. Promotional rates from 1-2% per transaction are not uncommon, and a 1% fee on a card with 1% cash back is a no-cost proposition. Point hackers take this to extremes using specific card perks to manufacture spending, but that's beyond the scope of this book.

Plastiq example:

- Delaying $10,000 in loans at 5% by 6 months saves $250.
- Paying a 2.5% charge on $10,000 also costs $250.

So, you'd break even between interest savings and the fee, but then you'd accrue points, miles, or the cash back on the card and thus end up on top.

Frankly, I think medical students probably have more important things to do than become point hackers. Even with the research and skill to master the craft, given that your entire life is probably financed, it will take serious diligence to use points to pay for expenses you can't avoid (paying for food staples or maybe traveling home for the holidays) and not to result in extra spending you would otherwise not have undertaken (trip to Europe). That being said, a service like Plastiq can help you reach the mandatory minimums on new cards to get the bonuses that make the whole endeavor worthwhile, particularly if your non-housing non-tuition life expenses are too small to qualify.

But, perhaps more importantly, the average medical student borrows way too much to be able to have enough cards to charge everything. Remember, the point is to have cards with 0% introductory rates. So, you'd have to get a new series of cards every semester or year depending on the various terms of the cards you get. Without much income and a fantastic credit history, getting enough to charge 40k+ a year probably isn't going to happen.

But you can probably get a new card periodically and charge a lot of your living expenses. Possibly your apartment, either directly or through Plastiq, but at least all of your meals, gas, consumer purchases, etc. The idea is to get a new card with a 0% introductory rate, charge as much of those expenses as you can (**but keep track so that you never ever go over your loan limits**), and then take out the loan money as late as possible in the semester to pay it all down. This is not an excuse to buy more stuff you don't need. To do this, you'll need to be extra diligent and responsible with your expenses. Credit card debt is much worse than student loan debt. If you're spending enough money to really bank on credit rewards, you're probably spending too much money.

Imagine someone who needs $40k a year in loans, $25k for tuition, $15k for living expenses. Usually, that $40k would come in two disbursements, one given at the beginning of each semester. Imagine you could delay each $7.5k for living by six months with credit cards. At 5.7%, each delay would be around $214, plus you'd get the points/cash back/perks from the credit card. So, you could shave off a couple thousand just by borrowing when you need the money and not just taking the full lump sum at the beginning just to let it sit around in your bank account doing nothing while the loan accrues interest. In practice, this also depends on how you pay for housing.

There are data showing that credit cards are psychologically dangerous. It's been demonstrated, for example, that people spend less money when they use cash instead of plastic. It all *feels* more real when it's paper in your hand. But, for a generally responsible person, credit cards are not the work of the devil: they're potentially dangerous tools of convenience.

But, in conclusion, I really don't believe that the more involved methods are a great idea for most students. However, the basic principle of not borrowing money until you need it is completely sound and recommended: there's no reason to borrow money to pay for a latte five months in advance.

CONSUMPTION SMOOTHING

Consumption smoothing is the idea that you borrow more now and spend less later to maintain a consistent lifestyle. This runs the risk of hedonic adaptation and lifestyle creep, but essentially everyone practices at least a mild form of this strategy. It's certainly what happens when you decide to use borrowed money to live somewhere nicer or drive something better than what is strictly necessary to survive.

The most important thing is that you don't inflate your lifestyle such that you are trying to live as an attending on a resident salary, living far beyond even your comparatively meager salary and paying no attention to the consequences of your spending and debt. Make no mistake: it's not the absolute values but the habits during residency that matter most. In the grand scheme of things, even doing the "wrong" thing with your loans during residency won't bankrupt you. But doing that as a first step to a lifetime of overspending and undersaving could easily do the trick.

You know what else will improve your lifetime finances? Marrying rich and never getting divorced. Obviously not everything in life is primarily a financial decision.

YOUR STUDENT LOAN "LIMIT"

It's generally considered undesirable to borrow more to finance an education than you can expect to earn in your first year's salary. That's because when someone borrows up to their first-year salary, it's generally doable to pay back their loans over a standard 10-year repayment. Borrow more and the cut on your investment return (in yourself) grows and grows. Ignoring residency, you've likely noticed that attending physicians have widely variable income. By this logic, those going into higher-paying specialties should have more leeway when it comes to borrowing for school. Perhaps not fair, but definitely true. Likewise, those considering poorly compensated specialties should be wary about attending expensive private schools unless willing to work at government or nonprofit institutions in order to receive public service loan forgiveness (PSLF). Since many students don't know what the future holds, a conservative borrowing outlook is the safest.

SO, PICK A HIGH-PAYING SPECIALTY?

I'll be the first person to tell you that you should pick something that makes you happy. But, medical school being imperfect, many medical students are still forced to ultimately guess at what specialties they would actually enjoy. What seems exciting and intellectually stimulating for a few weeks during a third-year clerkship might not feel the same after a few years. And then more years. Almost everything in medicine can become routine when you practice long enough, and every field has its pros/cons and layers of BS.

So, if you're *really* deciding between two specialties and it feels like a toss-up? Just pick the one with the better pay or lifestyle. If it makes you squeamish to have picked for money instead of some noble calling, just don't tell anyone. After a few years, I'm sure you'll be able to convince yourself it was because you *really loved the pathology.*

THE PURPOSE OF MONEY

Consider for yourself the true purpose of money: to allow you to live and to support your happiness. The "correct" financial decision from the "having more money is always better" perspective is always to pick that which costs the least amount of money or saves you the most. But most people don't live and can't live their lives exclusively in the service of accumulating dollars and cents. If that were the case, you may not have chosen to become a doctor in the first place, and many of you would not pick or have picked the specialties you did pick, some of which are considerably underpaid.

Consider that a few years of forbearance might cost that average-ish $200k borrower around $36,000 in unpaid capitalized interest during training and an extra $2,000 in annual interest over the long term: a considerable sum. Like a nice new car paid in cash. But that amount could also be the difference between you doing residency in a place that you love and that excites you instead of a place that doesn't; the difference between coming home to a relaxing evening in a place that you like after a long day at work or coming home after a long commute to a hovel. In many cases, the forbearance vs. loans decision won't hinge on these macro choices, but in others, you really have to sit down and think about your priorities. Residency can be hard enough as it is. If your future job has solid earning potential, who is to say taking a hit of tens of thousands of dollars is a *categorically wrong* choice?

(Forgive the upcoming cliché barrage)

Live like a student now or live like a student later. Live like a resident now or live like a resident later. Sometimes that can actually be true. How will your future self feel about your current self's decisions?

It depends on how you maximize utility. Some people are prodigious savers and get great satisfaction from putting money away for the future. That's great (it really is). But even if you have a hard time being thrifty, you should at least acknowledge that your future self already has plenty of things to pay for, including hopefully a long and healthy retirement. Don't forget that a penny saved is actually more than a penny earned (thanks to taxes).

But if spending some money now brings you great joy, I don't want to be a miser and imply that you can't spend some in an otherwise reasonable matter. Just don't forget that it's much easier to grow into your income than it is to deflate your lifestyle. You can always spend more money; it's very easy.

But it's very very hard to get off the hedonic treadmill.

In addition to eventually dealing with your student loans, there are several other things your money should also be earmarked for in the short term:

- Paying off any outstanding credit card debt. High-interest credit card debt is a financial emergency.

- An emergency fund (3-6 months of expenses in a safe place, say a free interest-bearing online savings account)

- Paying off any high-interest personal loans or other debt

- Appropriate insurance (disability, life) when you can afford it; get it while you're young. Generally, it's good to get this before finishing residency. If you have children, you need life insurance, period.

THE POWER OF INTEREST

WHAT IS INTEREST?

Interest is your source of pain as a debt holder and the purpose of investing. As a borrower, interest reflects your charge from lenders in order to use their money. It's also the source of their profits.

When you take out a loan, the balance is called the principal. When you borrow money, interest accrues on the principal based on the loan's interest rate, which is usually expressed as an annual percentage. A loan of $100,000 loan with a 5% interest rate accrues $5,000 a year. As we discussed, your medical school student loans begin accruing interest immediately when you get them, even while in school.

THE RULE OF 72

As a fun aside, the Rule of 72 is helpful shorthand to determine the approximate doubling time of an investment (or the doubling time of your loans while you're not making payments like when you're forbearing). Simply divide 72 by your interest rate: that's the number of years it will take. For example, at 6%, an investment (or unpaid loan) takes 12 years to double.

THE COST OF STARBUCKS

Personal finance gurus love to talk about the financial drag of a Starbucks habit on your budget/savings/you-name-it. It's on every top 10 list on every blog that has ever mentioned the word "money."

So, to pile on, let's consider the cost of a $4 Starbucks latte purchased with an unsubsidized loan during your first year of medical school with a 6.8% loan. After 4 years, it's now about $5.20. After a standard ten-year repayment, those four bucks you borrowed cost you $10. And *then* you still have to pay that $10 with after-tax money (so closer to $12-15 of earnings). Now it'd be less dramatic for coffees purchased with money held less long, and of course inflation reduces the effect a fair bit (a 2% inflation rate makes it about $7.70 once adjusted)—but it's still something to consider. When you borrow for tuition and cost of living, your entire life is a loan. The whole thing. You can cut coupons, but no matter the good deals you get, you may still end up paying double for every latte or burrito.

So even if this example is a bit silly, it does serve to illustrate the point: those loans may come easily, but they don't come cheap. And hey, if future-you wouldn't bat an eye at a $10 latte, then sip away.

COMPOUNDING/CAPITALIZATION

Compounding and capitalization are actually the same process, referred to as the "eighth wonder of the world" by none other than Albert Einstein. Capitalization occurs when accrued interest is added permanently to the principal, thus making the principal larger. That larger principal now grows interest faster than the original smaller amount. If this compounding happens on a regular basis, the loan grows faster and faster. This is the magic. As Benjamin Franklin said, "Interest never sleeps."

Compounding is what this phenomenon is called when referring to investment growth (a good thing), and capitalization is what it's called when it comes to debt (a bad thing).

To illustrate, imagine a $200,000 unsubsidized loan with a 5% interest rate after a one-year forbearance. The loan accrues $10,000 in interest (200,000 x .05) over the year. At the end of forbearance, the accrued interest is capitalized such that the new principal is $210,000. The loan now accrues $10,500 every year until payments are large enough to pay off the interest and start reducing the principal.

Since many residents' payments are not large enough to cover the accrued interest, that extra $500 per year from that one-year forbearance could happen for several years. Your loans capitalize at the end of your six-month grace period, so unless you have enough money to magically pay off all the interest that accrued while you were in school, you'll be feeling the effects of capitalization at least once.

As we mentioned in the above example, capitalization is one of the costs of choosing loan forbearance to avoid making payments. Most folks are limited to a three-year maximum, but as a trainee, you don't have that limit. You can be the proud recipient of the *mandatory medical residency forbearance*, which is mandatory in the sense that they are mandated to give it to you if you ask (not mandatory that you take it).

AMORTIZATION

Amortization is the process of how your loan is paid off gradually over a specified amount of time with the same size payment. Early on, the majority of your payments cover interest with a small amount applied to the principal. Over time though, the fraction of each payment going toward the loan itself continues to increase as the loan balance decreases and thus the daily interest decreases. This is exactly how mortgages work, and it explains why homeowners have very little equity in their homes for several years despite making what seem like large payments. Most of it is going to interest so that the bank can get its due.

NEGATIVE AMORTIZATION

Negative amortization is what happens when your monthly payments are insufficient to cover the accruing interest. Thus, despite making regular payments, the total amount owed continues to increase. This is a frustrating situation for borrowers, and in the context of medical student loans, very common during residency. That's because income-driven repayment plans cap your monthly payments at a reasonable level and your debt is frequently unreasonably large.

For example, a single resident with an AGI of $55,000 a year will have a monthly payment of around $308/month under the PAYE or REPAYE repayment plans, so about $3,700 a year. An average

$190,000 loan at 6% accrues $11,400 in interest per year, which means $7,700 would be unpaid. Despite what's felt to be an affordable monthly payment, that loan is only getting bigger. Negative amortization: Ouch.

FIXED VS VARIABLE RATES

All federal Direct loans are fixed rate, which means that the interest rate is set at the time of origination and will never change. You know exactly how much interest will accrue for a given loan amount over a given amount of time.

Private loans or privately refinanced loans can be fixed or variable. Variable-rate loans, like adjustable-rate mortgages, have rates that are tied to some external measure and can change over time. When the LIBOR (London Interbank Offered Rate)—or some other benchmark reflecting the rate that banks borrow from each other—goes up, your rate also goes up. This introduces some risk, and as a result, the offered rates are lower as an enticement. There's no free lunch. Whether or not that risk is worth it depends on several factors, including how much lower the variable rate is, how fast the rate can change, how fast you plan on paying off your loans, and how much faster you can pay them off if the rates increase rapidly. Interest rates are still basically at historic lows, but it's imprudent to make predictions about rate changes. It's like predicting the stock market. Anyone who is willing to tell you how to do it, if they really could, wouldn't be telling you. If as an attending you'll be making enough money that you could hunker down and pay your loans in a year or two, then the risk is negligible. If the ten-year standard is instead looking *just* on the cusp of doable, then it's probably better to stick with fixed.

LONGER REPAYMENT ALWAYS MEANS MORE COST

Interest doesn't have duty hours. The longer it takes you to pay off your loans, the more interest accrues, and the more interest you'll have to pay. When you pick a plan with lower payments and a longer repayment period, you also resign yourself to paying more money in the long run.

HOW STUDENT LOAN INTEREST ACTUALLY WORKS

While we often talk about annual interest, it's worth pointing out that federal student loan interest actually accrues daily. To determine your daily interest rate, divide the rate you have by 365. 6% APR is 0.0164% per day, so a $200,000 loan at 6% accrues about $33 a day in interest (200,000 x .000164) (more than your Starbucks and Chipotle by a long shot).

On the plus side, there is a 0.25% interest rate reduction when you auto-debit your monthly payments from your checking or savings account. So there's that. Once you're actually paying money every month, the rate will be a quarter point lower.

HOW MUCH DO YOU OWE (AND TO WHOM)?

Most people have exclusively federal loans.

Immediate Aside: If you *do* have any private loans, they are ineligible for all of the magical repayment plans and other possible forgiveness mumbo-jumbo that make up a big portion of this book. The best thing you can do with private loans is to make sure you have the lowest rate possible for the shortest term you can afford and then pay them off. There are a few options for private refinancing available to residents (discussed in the chapter on private refinance) and many more options available to attendings (due to their substantially superior income). If a company can offer you a better rate than the private loans you have currently, then refinance. Refinancing is a no-cost proposition and need not be avoided when it makes sense. For private loans, it's often a no-brainer. Refinance now, and if rates drop significantly, refinance again.

GET YOUR STUDENT DEBT SNAPSHOT:

Visit https://www.nslds.ed.gov and see how much you owe (this will show every cent you've borrowed from the feds and how much you currently owe on it). You'll also see who the servicers are for each loan if you have more than one.

If you have any private loans, you'll have to find those separately (if you can't keep track of them, they're on your credit report). You can also see your federal loans using the MedLoans calculator by logging into your AAMC account (which still works as a resident, in case you were curious), though the assumptions it uses to illustrate your options are inappropriate for anyone who is doing some serious planning. It'll give you a rough idea of what you'll be paying over the long term if you were to choose a repayment plan and stick with it forever.

NSLDS also gives you several more important bits of information:

What kind of loan?

If the lender is US Department of Education, it's a DIRECT loan and is eligible for all the IDR repayment plans. If you have some really old loans, they may have a different lender and won't be eligible for all the same plans.

Status: Deferment, In-school, Forbearance, Grace, Repayment

Also included are the current loan balance including principal and accrued interest, disbursement date, interest rate, servicer, etc.

CREATE YOUR VIRTUAL CONSOLIDATION

So now you have all of your loans laid out, each with their own interest rate. There may be times you want to have the granular data (particularly if you have a mix of federal and private loans), but if you haven't consolidated your loans, you'll likely want to create a "virtual" consolidation loan with a weighted average interest rate to in order to evaluate your options. To do this:

Add up all the loan balances including accrued interest. This is your new principal balance.

Multiply each loan's interest rate by its loan amount divided by your total loan amount. Add up all the weighted rates, and that's your weighted average.

(Note: this is exactly what happens when you do a federal direct consolidation loan.)

Arbitrary illustration:

- Loan 1: $50,000 at 6.8%

- Loan 2: $55,000 at 6.4%

- Loan 3: $60,000 at 6%

- Loan 4: $62,000 at 5.8%

Virtual consolidation:

Total: $227,000

Weighted Rate: .068 x 50/227 + .064 x 55/227 + .06 x 60/227 + .058 x 62/227 = .062

So, we're looking at $227,000 at an average interest rate of 6.2%.

There are free online calculators to do this simple math for you, like this one: https://www.doctoredmoney.org/student-debt/weighted-average-interest-rate-calculator

After this step, you now have the big (scary) numbers. Next, we'll discuss how federal loans work and what you can do about them.

HOW FEDERAL LOANS WORK

DIRECT & UNSUBSIDIZED

Nowadays, all federal student loans are lent directly by the federal government itself (so-called "Direct" loans). Prior to the financial crisis in 2008, loans were predominately given by private lenders/banks but "guaranteed" by the government under the now-defunct Federal Family Education Loan (FFEL) program. Direct loans are given out to undergraduate and graduates at different interest rates, and some of the undergraduate loans are subsidized so that they do not accrue interest while in school (this used to be true for graduate students as well until 2012).

Even though the loans are made by the government, the government itself has decided to not be directly responsible for *managing* all of them. They scut this duty of handling payments to several "servicers," including FedLoan, Nelnet, Navient, Great Lakes (the big four), MOHELA, CornerStone, Granite State, OSLA, and EdFinancial.

Unsubsidized student loans (the only kind of direct loan you can now get for medical school) begin accruing interest from the moment they are disbursed, so graduating students will already have a substantial amount of interest accrued on their original loan amounts. However, this in-school interest hasn't yet been capitalized (added to the principal loan balance). This interest eventually does capitalize at the end of grace period, unfortunately, so ultimately most residents will be looking at a loan that's bigger than the sum of the individual loans they took out every year. We'll talk plenty about this process later.

LOAN FEES

Loans fees (often called "origination fees") are subtracted from the loan disbursements, which means that you get less to spend than the amount you actually owe. The fee for Direct unsubsidized and subsidized loans are around 1%. For PLUS loans, the origination fee is around 4.27% (one reason why PLUS loans are an expensive proposition that should be avoided if possible).

Direct Loan Fees:

DIRECT SUBSIDIZED LOANS AND DIRECT UNSUBSIDIZED LOANS

2017-2018 (10/1/17 - 9/30/18)	1.066%
2016-2017 (10/1/16 - 9/30/17)	1.069%
2015-2016 (10/1/15 - 9/30/16)	1.068%
2014-2015 (10/1/14 - 9/30/15)	1.073%
2014-2015 (7/1/14 - 9/30/14)	1.072%
2013-2014 (12/1/13 - 6/30/14)	1.072%
2013-2014 (7/1/13 - 11/30/13)	1.051%
2012-2013 AND BEFORE	1.000%

DIRECT PLUS LOANS

2016-2017 (10/1/16 - 9/30/17)	4.276%
2015-2016 (10/1/15 - 9/30/16)	4.272%

DIRECT INTEREST RATES

Looking at your loans, you may notice that the rates aren't all the same. While all federal loans have a fixed rate (i.e. they don't change after you get them like a variable-rate loan will), the rates offered each year have changed annually as of 2013 after several years pegged at 6.8%. The annual rate is tied to the market rate of a 10-year Treasury note + a fixed margin (presumably what the government wants in profit). PLUS rates have recently been the graduate rate "plus" one.

RECENT DIRECT LOAN RATES

YEAR	UNDERGRADUATE SUB/UNSUB	GRADUATE UNSUB	PLUS
2017-18	4.45%	6.00%	7.00%
2016-17	3.76%	5.31%	6.31%
2015-16	4.29%	5.84%	6.84%
2014-15	4.66%	6.21%	7.21%
2013-14	3.86%	5.41%	6.41%
2012-13	3.40%	6.80%	7.90%
2011-12	4.50%	6.80%	7.90%
2010-11	5.60%	6.80%	7.90%
2009-10	6.00%	6.80%	7.90%
2008-09	6.80%	6.80%	7.90%

While recent medical students have lost the chance of even a dime of subsidized loans outside of the much smaller Perkins program, the interest rates on their debt have decreased significantly. It's still worth noting that all of these rates are still relatively high compared to the Fed's interest rate, which had been at the historic low of zero for several years until December 2016. Since overall interest rates have increased, the Direct rates are on the rise again and are back up to 6% for the 2017-2018 school year. Unless the economy nosedives, it would seem unlikely that rates will improve much in the near future.

The rates for undergrads are substantially lower (3.76% in 2016-17; 4.45% in 2017-18).

A Direct Consolidation loan has an interest rate that is a weighted average of its source loans, rounded up to the nearest 1/8 of 1% (0.125).

Also, note that the Direct sticker rate only really accrues when in-school or during forbearance. Once in repayment, you are eligible for a 0.25% reduction if you use autopay to debit your monthly payments. The feds tell you the true rate, but private companies will always show you their rate *with* the auto-debit discount. Make sure to compare apples to apples.

FEDERAL REPAYMENT OPTIONS

There are several repayment options available for federal student loans: traditional plans (standard, graduated, extended) and income-driven plans (income-based repayment (IBR), income-contingent repayment (ICR), pay as you earn (PAYE), and revised pay as you earn (REPAYE)). The plans are not one-time binding decisions, and you can switch plans if your needs or wants change as long as you still meet the eligibility criteria (if any).

If you consolidate at the end of school, you will also choose a repayment plan for the new consolidation loan at that time.

Otherwise, your servicer will contact you 1-2 months before your grace period ends to have you select a repayment plan. If you don't select anything, you will automatically be placed in the "Standard" plan.

Sample monthly payments for a single resident with a $200k loan at 6% with a $55,000 AGI:

Repayment Plan	Monthly Payment
Standard	$2,220
Graduated	$1,270
Extended	$1,289
Revised Pay As You Earn (REPAYE)	$308
Pay As You Earn (PAYE)	$308
Income-Based Repayment (IBR)	$461

STANDARD

The "standard" repayment is a 10-year repayment plan and technically the default option, though few residents will use it. If you don't select one of the other plans before the end of your grace period, you'll automatically be placed in the standard repayment plan. Monthly payments are set at the beginning of repayment and won't change. A student graduating with $200k of debt is looking at roughly $2,200/month for the standard repayment (i.e. ain't going to happen on a resident salary). Under the standard plan, you will pay off your loans after 10 years/120 payments.

While we'll keep referring to the 10-year Standard, note that for Direct Consolidation loans, the Standard plan is actually extended between 10-30 years depending on your loan amount, with 10 years for loans less than $7,500 and 30 years for amounts greater than $60,000. See: https://studentaid.ed.gov/sa/repay-loans/understand/plans/standard#monthly-payments-consolidation.

THE GRADUATED AND EXTENDED REPAYMENT PLANS

The graduated and extended plans are older pre-IDR-era plans largely irrelevant to current borrowers. Graduated repayment was designed for those who anticipate steadily increasing income, and monthly payments start low and then gradually increase every two years. The repayment term is generally 10 years, except for consolidation loans, which are stretched out to 30. The extended plan stretches out a stable monthly payment over 25 years. The various IDR programs are basically universally better options and have essentially supplanted both of these programs. You can essentially forget they exist, because if none of the IDR will work for you, then you should probably be on the standard 10-year plan or refinance.

INCOME-DRIVEN REPAYMENT PLANS (IDR)

IDR is an umbrella term generally used to refer to the big three: IBR, PAYE, and REPAYE. All of these plans tie your monthly payments to a percentage of your income and are recalculated on an annual basis.

You can apply for an IDR plan toward the end of your grace period or after consolidating your loans (more on that later). Your monthly payment is generally calculated using your tax returns. If your tax returns don't reflect your current income (e.g. when your taxes reflect you being a broke student but you're actually a slightly less broke intern), then you can (or may be forced to) use pay stubs or an employment letter/contract to demonstrate income. This ability can be also used to your advantage to reduce your monthly payment if your income decreases.

All IDR plans calculate your monthly payments based on your *discretionary income*. Your discretionary income is defined as your adjusted gross income minus 150% of the poverty line for your family size and state of residence. Your adjusted gross income (AGI) is your total income (wages, salaries, interest, dividends, etc.) minus "above the line" deductions like pretax retirement contributions. The AGI is reported on your federal income tax return, so you don't have to try to calculate it yourself. The poverty line depends on family size (and is also higher in Alaska and Hawaii).

In 2017, the federal poverty limits for the lower 48 states:

- $12,060 for individuals
- $16,240 for a family of 2
- $20,420 for a family of 3
- $24,600 for a family of 4
- $28,780 for a family of 5
- $32,960 for a family of 6
- $37,140 for a family of 7
- $41,320 for a family of 8

A single person's discretionary income in 2017 would be AGI - $18,090 (because 1.5 x 12,060 = 18,090).

Note that any repayment estimator/calculator will calculate your discretionary income from your AGI in order to generate IDR payment examples for you based on the information you provide, but it's helpful to know if you want to do any hand calculations (and to understand how the whole thing works). As you can see, every person in your family increases the poverty line by about $4,000 and reduces your AGI by about $6,000 (1.5 x $4,000, see IDR equations below).

Your ability to initially qualify for IBR and PAYE depends on if you have a **partial financial hardship (PFH)**. A PFH is when your calculated standard 10-year repayment exceeds 10 or 15% of your discretionary income. Put another way, if your calculated IBR or PAYE payment is less than the 10-year standard, then you have a PFH and qualify. As a quick rule of thumb, your AGI needs to be greater than your student loan balance when you entered repayment for you to not have a PFH (around 130% actually), an uncommon scenario for a resident. You'll need to submit your income certification annually. Even if your income goes up and you no longer have a PFH, you still stay in your IDR plan as long you as you recertify your income annually.

If you don't recertify, you don't get to stay on your current plan: From IBR or PAYE, you'll get punted to the standard 10-year plan. From REPAYE, you'll be placed on the "alternative" plan, which is functionally equivalent to the standard for most folks. If you try to switch plans, the greater of your initial repayment balance or your current balance is used for the PFH calculation.

All IDR plans pay 100% of the *unpaid* interest on *subsidized* loans (which you might have from your undergraduate days) for three years.

INCOME-BASED REPAYMENT (IBR)

IBR was the original "new" plan back in 2009 and the first plan eligible for PSLF. IBR limits monthly payments to 15% of discretionary income for those with a "partial financial hardship," and payments are capped at the Standard 10-year amount if income rises sufficiently. Both DIRECT and older FFEL loans qualify (but not Parent PLUS or any consolidation that included a Parent PLUS loan). The government will pay off any unpaid interest on subsidized loans for the first three years. Any remaining loans are forgiven after 25 years of payments (but the forgiven amount is subject to taxes—ouch).

Monthly payment: (AGI – 1.5 x poverty level) x 0.15 / 12 = IBR

IBR FOR NEW BORROWERS

"IBR for new borrowers" is just essentially an automatic way to phase out the old IBR program in favor of the newer PAYE. IBR for new borrowers (first loan from July 1, 2014, and beyond) changes the old IBR terms to the terms for PAYE, except for the lack of the cap on capitalized interest. There's really no reason to pick IBR if you are eligible for PAYE; please just pick PAYE.

PAYE

PAYE is analogous to IBR but with better terms: payments are calculated at 10% of discretionary income for those with a PFH (but again never more than the Standard 10-year amount). Forgiveness timeline is reduced to 20 years. Additionally, any capitalized interest (say after losing your PFH) is limited to 10% of the original principal amount upon entering repayment (potentially limiting a bit of needless suffering). The 3-year subsidized loan interest subsidy is the same.

Why doesn't everyone do PAYE instead of IBR then? Because PAYE is limited to DIRECT loan borrowers with no loans before October 1, 2007, AND with a new loan after October 1, 2011. Most current students these days *do* qualify for PAYE.

Monthly payment: (AGI − 1.5 x poverty level) x .10 / 12 = REPAYE or PAYE.

REPAYE

The newest kid on the block, released at the end of 2015: REPAYE was designed to extend the lower payments of PAYE to more borrowers (the IBR crowd) and provide relief from negative amortization while also closing some loopholes to limit costs. Payments are 10% of your discretionary income, period. You don't need a partial financial hardship to qualify, but the payments are never capped either: they continue to climb as you make money (potentially bad for PSLF, otherwise not necessarily an issue). In addition to the built-in IDR-wide 3-year subsidized loan interest subsidy we discussed previously, REPAYE also pays 50% of the unpaid interest on your *un-subsidized* loans as well forever starting day 1 (and 50% on your sub-sidized loans too after three years). Depending on the size of your loans (and the size of your payments), this can be a lot of money, and it effectively lowers your interest rate. In addition to the remov-al of the payment cap, the "married filing separately" loophole is closed (discussed in the PAYE vs REPAYE chapter), which primarily affects borrowers with high-earning low-debt spouses.

INCOME-CONTINGENT REPAYMENT (ICR)

ICR was the original IDR plan, way back in 1993. It's only relevant for people who need to pay off Parent PLUS loans (PLUS loans made to your parents), which are IBR/PAYE & PSLF ineligible but *are* ICR-eli-gible once placed into a Direct Consolidation Loan and were made after July 1, 2006. ICR can be dependent on income or loan amount: payments are the lesser of 20% of discretionary income or whatever amount would be required to pay off the loan over 12 years multiplied by a small "income factor" (which for residents will be around 1; see https://www.federalregister.gov/documents/2016/04/04/2016-07517/ annual-updates-to-the-income-contingent-repayment-icr-plan-formula-for-2016-william-d-ford-federal). 25-year forgiveness is available like IBR. Most young people can forget this exists.

Note for parents hoping to get PSLF on their consolidated Parent PLUS loans: it is *your* work and on-time monthly payments over ten years that matter for PSLF (not the dependent child who actual-ly went to school). Source: https://studentaid.ed.gov/sa/repay-loans/ forgiveness-cancellation/public-service/questions.

There is a loophole for parents hoping to get their Parent PLUS loans into a better repayment plan referred to as "Double Consol-idation," whereby the initial consolidation makes the loans eligible for ICR and then reconsolidating that consolidation loan somehow magically makes the government forget that the original consoli-dation was for a Parent PLUS loan in the first place. It's a little extra complicated because you can only consolidate the easy online way once at studentloans.gov.

The idea is that you file two paper applications by writing down your loan numbers from NSLDS by hand (scary!) to create two different consolidation loans with two different servicers and then go online and file for a new Direct consolidation loan combining the original two consolidation loans. Voilà.

INCOME-SENSITIVE REPAYMENT (ISR)

Completely irrelevant. This was originally an ICR alternative for people with old non-DIRECT loans made under the Federal Family Education Loan (FFEL) program, which was replaced and then finally terminated in 2010. IBR essentially replaced ISR entirely. The monthly loan payment was pegged to a fixed percentage of gross monthly income (not adjusted gross income like the other IDR plans), between 4% and 25%, which is chosen by the borrower but *must be greater than or equal to the accrued interest*. Very unique. Unlike the other plans, you can only be in ISR for up to 5 years.

Unless you're a nontraditional student who finished undergraduate studies a long time ago, you probably don't have any FFEL loans (which if you do are—to repeat—eligible for IBR, just not PAYE or REPAYE). Again, you can check National Student Loan Data System (NSLDS) to see who owns your loans.

LOAN ELIGIBILITY TABLE

LOAN TYPE	REPAYE PLAN	PAYE PLAN	IBR PLAN	ICR PLAN
DIRECT SUBSIDIZED LOANS	Yes	Yes	Yes	Yes
DIRECT UNSUBSIDIZED LOANS	Yes	Yes	Yes	Yes
DIRECT PLUS LOANS MADE TO STUDENTS	Yes	Yes	Yes	Yes
DIRECT PLUS LOANS MADE TO PARENTS	Never	Never	Never	If Consolidated
DIRECT CONSOLIDATION LOANS	Yes	Yes	Yes	Yes
DIRECT CONSOLIDATION LOANS *THAT INCLUDE A PARENT PLUS LOAN*	Never	Never	Never	Yes
SUBSIDIZED FEDERAL STAFFORD LOANS (FFEL)	If Consolidated	If Consolidated	Yes	If Consolidated
UNSUBSIDIZED FEDERAL STAFFORD LOANS (FFEL)	If Consolidated	If Consolidated	Yes	If Consolidated
FFEL PLUS LOANS MADE TO STUDENTS	If Consolidated	If Consolidated	Yes	If Consolidated
FFEL PLUS LOANS MADE TO PARENTS	Never	Never	Never	If Consolidated

FFEL CONSOLIDATION LOANS	If Consolidated	If Consolidated	Yes	If Consolidated
FFEL CONSOLIDATION LOANS *THAT INCLUDE A PARENT PLUS LOAN*	Never	Never	Never	If Consolidated
FEDERAL PERKINS LOANS	If Consolidated	If Consolidated	If Consolidated	If Consolidated

As you can see, most new graduates' loans automatically qualify for any of the plans you'd actually want to use, and most that don't become so once consolidated. The exception is the Parent PLUS loan, which ruins everything.

And here's an example of how much a resident or fellow might expect to pay monthly as they advance through training:

MONTHLY IDR PAYMENTS BY YEAR*

REPAYMENT YEAR	CERTIFICATION TAX YEAR	COMPOSITE SALARY	PAYE/ REPAYE	IBR
PGY1	MS3-MS4	$0	$0	$0
PGY2	MS4-PGY1	$27,500	$78	$118
PGY3	PGY1-2	$56,000	$316	$474
PGY4	PGY2-3	$58,000	$333	$499
PGY5	PGY3-4	$60,000	$349	$524
PGY6	PGY4-5	$62,000	$366	$549
PGY7	PGY5-6	$64,000	$383	$574
PGY8	PGY6-7	$66,000	$399	$599

*Assuming an intern salary of $55,000, increasing by $2,000 annually with repayment starting in July using tax returns for income certification. Each calendar repayment year is based on two academic years: the second half of one with the first half of the next.

Here is an illustration of how IDR payments scale with household income in the continental US. The more you make, the closer it gets to being 10/15% as income grows relative to the poverty level:

IDR PAYMENTS BY HOUSEHOLD INCOME

AGI	MONTHLY PAYE/ REPAYE	ANNUAL PAYE/ REPAYE	MONTHLY IBR	ANNUAL IBR
$50,000	$266	$3,192	$399	$4,788
$55,000	$308	$3,696	$461	$5,532
$60,000	$349	$4,188	$524	$6,282
$65,000	$391	$4,692	$586	$7,032
$70,000	$433	$5,196	$649	$7,788
$75,000	$474	$5,688	$711	$8,532
$80,000	$516	$6,192	$774	$9,288
$90,000	$599	$7,188	$899	$10,782
$100,000	$683	$8,196	$1,024	$12,288
$110,000	$766	$9,192	$1,149	$13,788
$120,000	$849	$10,188	$1,274	$15,282
$130,000	$933	$11,196	$1,399	$16,788

$140,000	$1,016	$12,192	$1,524	$18,288
$150,000	$1,099	$13,188	$1,649	$19,782
$160,000	$1,183	$14,196	$1,774	$21,288
$170,000	$1,266	$15,192	$1,899	$22,788
$180,000	$1,349	$16,188	$2,024	$24,282
$190,000	$1,433	$17,196	$2,149	$25,788
$200,000	$1,516	$18,192	$2,274	$27,288
$220,000	$1,683	$20,196	$2,524	$30,288
$240,000	$1,849	$22,188	$2,774	$33,282
$260,000	$2,016	$24,192	$3,024	$36,288
$280,000	$2,183	$26,196	$3,274	$39,288
$300,000	$2,349	$28,188	$3,524	$42,282
$350,000	$2,766	$33,192	$4,149	$49,788
$400,000	$3,183	$38,196	$4,774	$57,288
$450,000	$3,599	$43,188	$5,399	$64,782
$500,000	$4,016	$48,192	$6,024	$72,288

FEDERAL REPAYMENT LOGISTICAL CONSIDERATIONS

SHADY HELP

You don't need a company to help you enter or change your payment plan or "qualify" for forgiveness. These are scams. Picking or switching repayment plans is free and only takes a few minutes online.

YOU CAN'T JUST DIRECTLY PAY OFF THE PRINCIPAL

Unlike your mortgage or many other loans, you can't just apply extra payments directly to the loan principal. The servicer must put any extra payments toward interest first. Given the negative amortization scenario most residents find themselves in (and which fuels the REPAYE subsidy), making extra payments isn't going to help you reduce your principal/slow your rate of interest growth (it'll reduce the actual amount of interest accruing, but making payments toward principal would allow less to accrue per unit time in the first place). Until you pay off all the accrued interest, you can't dent the principal.

AUTO-DEBIT RATE REDUCTION

You do get an automatic 0.25% interest rate reduction once you begin auto-pay (auto-debiting monthly payments from your checking or savings account).

Note this only happens when you're auto-paying a non-zero amount, so if you have a calculated zero payment, you don't get the rate reduction. You can't ask to make a $5 payment and get the benefit; it's only once your required payment is more than $0.

SWITCHING PLANS

You can always switch plans to any plan for which you are eligible. This means that you can always switch to Standard and REPAYE (which have no eligibility requirements) and can switch into IBR or

PAYE when you meet the above criteria (e.g. partial financial hardship). Remember, if you try to switch plans, the greater of your initial repayment balance or your current loan balance is used for the PFH calculation. Just because your loans may be getting smaller doesn't mean you don't have a PFH.

CAPITALIZATION TRIGGERS

The following are events that trigger capitalization:

- End of grace period / beginning of repayment

- End of a period of forbearance or deferment

- Change repayment plan or consolidation

- Loss of partial financial hardship in IBR or PAYE

- Failure to submit IDR annual income certification on time

- Loan Default

DEALING WITH SERVICERS

It's very important to talk to your servicer and make sure that everybody is on the same page and your plans will work out the way they're supposed to. It's also very important not to simply take the phone representatives' word if what they're saying seems wrong or doesn't make sense with everything you've learned elsewhere. The servicer folks are "free" customer service representatives, not experts in finance or even experts about their own services. Frequently, they are misinformed about the details and nuances of what is and is not allowed. Whether they're being willfully ignorant or deliberately obtuse, servicers are notorious for saying things that are simply not true. You may need to be prepared to fight if you plan anything creative, particularly when it comes to switching plans and getting your loans forgiven.

If you're dissatisfied, you can file an official complaint via the Federal Student Aid Feedback System: https://feedback.studentaid.ed.gov/.

They will attempt to resolve the issue within 60 days.

If your servicer is being evil or dishonest and you can't get them to see reason and your complaint didn't work out, you can enlist the help of a federal student loan ombudsmen, a free last resort offered by the US Department of Education. The Federal Student Aid (FSA) Ombudsman Group is an impartial third party that may be able to help resolve issues, but they aren't guaranteed to be on your side. You can read more info about it here if you're curious or need to: https://studentaid.ed.gov/sa/repay-loans/disputes/prepare.

Many borrowers have had good luck filing a complaint with the Consumer Finance Protection Bureau (CFPB), especially with repeated miscounting of qualifying payments by FedLoan with regard to PSLF: https://www.consumerfinance.gov/complaint/

INCOME-DRIVEN REPAYMENT

As we've discussed, there are multiple loan repayment programs available, but the vast majority of borrowers are eligible for and will choose an IDR plan during residency. Those with lower loan amounts and no partial financial hardship should instead go with the standard plan, which will spread out your complete repayment over 10 years, or refinance privately. Outside of loan forgiveness, never forget that you can and often should pay your loans off faster than the plan will schedule if you can afford it.

For practical purposes, the other plans mentioned in the last chapter can be safely ignored: for typical residents who easily have a partial financial hardship, it's overall better to pick one of the main three IDR plans (IBR, PAYE, or REPAYE) and make extra payments than it is to pick the extended or graduated plans, which have no associated benefits.

Traditional loan repayment is based on a length of time. IDR is based on a percentage of income (hence "income-driven"). It's important to realize that IDR is designed to make your loan payments affordable and NOT to "save you money." Setting and forgetting an IDR plan will not generate payments that reflect how much money you could really afford to pay on your loans, particularly as your income increases, and thus will not pay down your loans in the timeliest (and thus cheapest) way possible.

If you're trying to get your loans forgiven, then minimizing payments will save you money (no point spending dollars toward something you ultimately won't be accountable for). But if you need to actually pay off your loans, which applies to a lot of people, making lower payments can mean taking longer to pay off your loans and more money wasted on interest (we'll discuss how the REPAYE interest subsidy temporarily changes that for many residents in the REPAYE chapter).

GENERAL CONSIDERATIONS FOR ALL IDR PLANS

The oft-reported "downside" of income-driven repayment plans is that you will "pay more interest" over the inevitably longer term length. This is a bit misleading, because you are always free to send in more money to pay off your loan faster. The longer it takes you to pay your loans down, the more money you waste on interest. But it doesn't mean that an IDR plan isn't the right selection.

IDR plans allow you the flexibility to not need to make big payments and to qualify for loan forgiveness in the future; they don't prevent you from taking prudent measures to pay down your debt.

BREAKING EVEN

It's helpful to know what your break-even rate is, which is the rate at which your calculated IDR payments match interest accrual. You're making no progress, but your debt isn't growing either. Determine your monthly interest: loan amount multiplied by interest rate divided by 12. That's basically your accruing monthly interest (technically that would be the daily interest rate times the number of days in the month, but you get the idea).

Then, go the calculator and adjust the AGI field until the first monthly payment under your plan of choice is the same thing. This is basically the salary you'll need to contain negative amortization. It's probably more than you'll ever make as a resident.

Here's an illustrative breakdown of the break-even AGI for different loan amounts at 6%:

SALARY NEEDED TO MATCH ACCRUING INTEREST IN IDR

LOAN AMOUNT	ANNUAL INTEREST (6%)	MONTHLY	PAYE/ REPAYE AGI	IBR AGI
$100,000	$6,000	$500	$78,000	$58,000
$150,000	$9,000	$750	$108,000	$78,000
$200,000	$12,000	$1,000	$138,000	$98,000
$250,000	$15,000	$1,250	$168,000	$118,000
$300,000	$18,000	$1,500	$198,000	$138,000
$350,000	$21,000	$1,750	$228,000	$158,000
$400,000	$24,000	$2,000	$258,000	$178,000
$450,000	$27,000	$2,250	$288,000	$198,000
$500,000	$30,000	$2,500	$318,000	$218,000

These rounded rough estimates illustrate three important things. One, it takes a pretty solid income for a lot of folks to just *break even* on an IDR plan. While IBR and PAYE max out at the standard repayment, even many attendings will never hit that cap.

Second, large borrowers could easily drown without programs like PSLF. Someone who owes $400,000 would need a salary of over $250k just to have their calculated monthly payments match the rate of interest accumulation. While they could certainly pay more money and make some progress, it's not a heartening prospect.

Lastly, the break-even salary is also the salary at which all accruing interest is paid and thus there are no unpaid interest subsidies. The effective rate equals the real rate. We'll talk more about this in a minute.

OVERPAYMENT CAN BE A GOOD THING

The technical downside of picking a plan with the lowest monthly payments is that, if followed, you will pay your loan over a longer period of time and thus pay more interest over the terms of your loan. You'll see this on every chart and table, but it's a bit of an artificial construct for doctors, whose income is likely to change significantly over the course of repayment. Picking a plan with low payments does not mean you're obligated to only pay at that lower amount forever. For example, a resident may pick a low payment during residency and then step up and blast their debt as an attending. This often discussed "downside" of IDR only applies to picking a plan beneath what you can really afford and then never reevaluating. Once you can afford more, pay more.

PSLF CHANGES EVERYTHING

Keep in mind the plus/minus of different plans depends very much on whether or not we're trying to minimize the total amount of money it takes you to pay off your loans (a generally good idea) or if we're trying to minimize payments in order to not waste money before achieving loan forgiveness (also a good idea). We'll discuss PSLF in depth in a bit.

While it's technically correct to generally pay down your highest interest rate debt first, this does not apply to people who are considering public service loan forgiveness. Even if your car payment has a lower interest rate than your student loans, you may be better off investing for your retirement (tax savings and PSLF implications are great) or paying down a car note (thus improving monthly cash flow), because extra loan payments will just reduce the windfall you'll receive if you achieve PSLF. Paying off smaller debts like cars also ties into the "debt snowball" method, where you tackle your smallest debt amounts first instead of your highest interest, which enables you to reduce the number of different things you owe money on and psychologically feels awesome.

MARRIAGE CONSIDERATIONS

Double income + double federal loans are treated essentially like a single income single loan when it comes to calculating IDR. The total loans are grouped, and your income is pooled. The total amount owed is calculated and each person pays an amount to their loans weighted to their individual contribution to the total loan amount. As in, if one spouse owes $200k and one owes $100k and the calculated payment is $999, then one spouse will pay $666 and the other $333.

There is a "married filing separately" loophole in IBR and PAYE: if you file your taxes separately from your spouse, you can shield their income from the IDR calculation. Each spouse is then treated as if they were a single unmarried individual with their individual debt and individual income. Trying to file separately to reduce payments can be helpful if you're going for forgiveness or have cash flow problems and need the money to spend. The classic scenario to file separately is one graduating medical student with tons of debt and one high-earning spouse with none. Note that REPAYE closed this loophole, so if this trick is critical to your plans, you'll need to switch out of the plan or not pick it in the first place.

There are tax consequences to filing separately, and you lose out on some deductions. You can calculate your taxes both ways using tax software (or with your accountant) to see how much it'll cost you and if the savings in IDR payments are worth it. If both spouses are going for PSLF, don't bother filing separately. And if you're not going for PSLF at all then filing separately is just another way to lower payments but consequently prolong the agony.

Lastly, if one spouse refinances privately, their loans are no longer eligible for IDR. Thus, for REPAYE (or for IBR/PAYE when you file taxes jointly), the remaining party with federal loans will see a big payment increase, because suddenly the household income is unchanged but the "total" loan amount will be reduced. In the above example, imagine the $100k spouse refinances. Now that same

$999 payment calculated from their joint income is due just for the $200k loan. Meanwhile, the refinanced $100k loan still has its own payment. Outside of loan forgiveness, you don't *lose* money this way, but you do end up spending more per month.

ANNUAL INCOME CERTIFICATION

Borrowers generally certify their income by submitting their most recent tax return. What that means in practice is that you're actually using *last year's* income to calculate the coming year's payments.

As in, when you certify your income in 2017 to make payments for 2017-18, you'll use your *2016* tax return. There is a built-in lag between any income changes and when they have an effect on your payments. That is, unless you check the little box on the form saying that your income has *decreased* substantially compared with what's reflected in your tax returns (it used to say "changed," but this was clarified in 2019).

Don't certify early most years, as it will generally only increase your payments faster (because your resident income goes up a bit every year). But if your income goes down or your family size is going up, consider recertifying immediately. Just be aware that you'll often be asked for evidence of your *current income* (i.e. pay stubs) as opposed to your previously filed *adjusted gross income*. If you utilize retirement contributions or other tax deductions, it's possible that you can actually raise payments this way because even though your income has gone down, it may still be higher than your AGI was after all was said and done.

If your adjusted gross income is going to increase a lot and you want to change plans before it's reflected in your new tax returns, you can try to recertify early and change plans before it's too late.

Also note that you should account for unborn children in your family size, so if you recertify in July and your first child is due in December, your family size is three instead of two.

If you are late in submitting your annual certification, it will cause an automatic interest capitalization. Don't be late. The servicer generally will but is not obligated to contact you, so put it on your calendar.

If you lose your PFH at certification time, your interest will capitalize in IBR and PAYE, but you will *never* be kicked out of the plan. If you receive a confusing letter in the mail saying you "no longer qualify," it's just a poorly-worded letter. Once in IBR, always in IBR. Once in PAYE, always in PAYE.

REPAYE

REPAYE (Revised Pay as You Earn) became the newest federal student loan repayment option at the end of 2015. Because of how REPAYE handles unpaid interest (negative amortization), it's the ideal plan for many (but not all) residents, even those who would otherwise qualify for PAYE.

LET'S REVIEW: WHAT IS REPAYE?

REPAYE was created to give older borrowers from the (pre-PAYE) IBR regime a chance to benefit from some features of the newer PAYE plan (payments based on 10% of your discretionary income instead of 15% in IBR) while also closing some of its "loopholes." As a general rule, the feds don't change current programs; they create new ones and "grandfather" people in the old ones. Rather than extending PAYE to more people (those with loans prior to October 1, 2007, or without new loans since October 1, 2011), they made REPAYE.

Here are the main features of the REPAYE program (contrasted with PAYE and IBR as applicable and how they may affect switching):

GOOD: 10% AGI PAYMENTS

Monthly payments are calculated at 10% of discretionary income (adjusted gross income minus the poverty line). If you're currently in IBR, this effectively cuts your monthly payment by 33%, saving you a good chunk per month and potentially saving you a lot over the course of the 10-year PSLF mark. If you're in PAYE, the monthly payment will be the same (with some exceptions outlined below).

GOOD: THE 50% UNPAID-INTEREST SUBSIDY

Subsidized loans for medical students are a thing of the past, but the new REPAYE program has actually added back a much more robust interest subsidy. In fact, the subsidy is the main feature that makes staying with federal loans during residency a reasonable alternative to private refinancing if you're otherwise not planning on trying to achieve PSLF.

The deal is this: half of the interest you don't pay with the calculated 10% payment is waived and does not accrue. This is a huge perk of the program and should cause even residents currently in PAYE to run some numbers, as it effectively reduces your interest rate while in training (in many cases to an effective rate lower than what private companies are able to match). For example, a $0 monthly payment reduces your interest rate by half(!).

An example:

- Loan: $200,000 at 6%
- REPAYE payment as a single resident making $55,000: $308/month
- Annual interest accrued: $12,000
- Annual interest paid: $3,696
- Annual interest unpaid: $8,304
- Amount forgiven: $4,152
- Remaining unpaid interest: $4,152
- Total annual interest: $7,848 (the amount you paid + the unpaid amount not forgiven)
- Effective interest rate: **3.92%**

The more you make, the higher your payment and thus the less interest unpaid and forgiven.

The more you owe, the greater the amount of interest remains unpaid and the more forgiven.

EFFECTIVE INTEREST RATES UNDER REPAYE (LOAN: $200,000 AT 6%)

SALARY	INTEREST PAID	INTEREST UNPAID	INTEREST FORGIVEN	EFFECTIVE ANNUAL INTEREST	EFFECTIVE RATE
$0	$0	$12,000	$6,000	$6,000	3.00%
$25,000	$696	$11,304	$5,652	$6,348	3.18%
$50,000	$3,192	$8,808	$4,404	$7,596	3.80%
$75,000	$5,688	$6,312	$3,156	$8,844	4.42%
$100,000	$8,196	$3,804	$1,902	$10,098	5.05%
$125,000	$10,692	$1,308	$654	$11,346	5.67%
$138,100	$12,000	$0	$0	$12,000	6.00%

In this example, once your monthly payment hits $1,000, you're breaking even with interest and nothing is forgiven (for a single physician, this corresponds to an annual income of around $138k, so sadly very much in the realm of some academic faculty jobs). Ultimately, this makes REPAYE the correct choice for even most non-PSLF-bound residents.

For attendings (or married residents) with a household income above the break-even point *not considering* PSLF, private refinancing will likely supply a better rate and more savings. Obviously, the more you owe, the more interest accrues, and the higher you have to earn before you break even on monthly interest. You really need to run your numbers! Private college + medical school and suddenly that subsidy could be good forever.

Of course, like IBR and PAYE, the unpaid interest you have on any subsidized loans (i.e. from college) is still completely covered for 3 years (and then 50% after that, like unsubsidized loans).

BAD: THE MARRIED-FILING-SEPARATELY "LOOPHOLE" IS CLOSED

REPAYE closes the married-filing-separately loophole. Under PAYE and IBR, if your spouse made big bucks, you could file taxes separately, thus calculating your loan payments for your debt based solely on your (lower) income. This was particularly helpful for doctors, especially low-earning residents, with high earning spouses who didn't have big student loans themselves. If you rely on exploiting the income disparity between you and your spouse to make income-driven repayment work for you, then you don't want to switch to REPAYE.

That said, if you and your spouse both have loans and similar income (i.e. both went to medical school around the same time and finished residency around the same time), then this isn't an issue. If you file together despite higher loan payments due to other tax benefits, you aren't using the loophole anyway. For example, you can only deduct student loan interest if you file jointly (but this deduction is unimpressively capped at $2,500 and only for households earning less than $165,000 in 2017). Run the payments both ways, and if it's a big difference, then check the tax costs.

BAD: THE PAY CAP IS GONE

REPAYE did away with the monthly payment cap. IBR payments are calculated at 15% of your discretionary income and PAYE payments are 10%, but both are capped at the monthly amount calculated by the standard 10-year repayment when you first entered repayment. So even if your salary as an attending is huge, your monthly payments could only rise so much (often referred to as the "Doctor's Loophole" due to the big salary jump at attendinghood with only a subdued concomitant rise in loan payments). There is no payment cap with REPAYE; your monthly payments keep scaling with income. For some, the IBR/PAYE cap is critical to potentially achieving PSLF, because if your income grows high enough fast enough you could "overpay" quickly and whittle down the forgiven amount. Practically, this change may be less important than it seems. It's all about the ratio of your loan amount to your income. The bigger your loan and the smaller your income, the less relevant this becomes. You can plug different incomes into the feds' calculator to run your numbers.

As a quick rule, you definitely need to make more per year than you owed at repayment for this to matter at all. So if you borrowed $200k and are making $150k doing primary care: probably irrelevant (depending on your spouse's income). You'll have to do your own numbers, but here's an example:

Loan amount: $200,000
Loan rate: 6.8%
Payments with annual income: $50,000

- IBR: $404

- PAYE: $270

- REPAYE: $270

- Standard: $2302

Payments with annual income: $250,000

- IBR: Capped at standard, $2302

- PAYE: $1936

- REPAYE: $1936

- Standard: $2302

Payments with annual income: $300,000

- IBR: Capped at standard, $2302

- PAYE: Capped at standard, $2302

- REPAYE: $2352

- Standard: $2302

As you can see, in this example it takes an income of nearly $300,000 for the uncapped REPAYE to finally cost more per month. For the average single doc, the cap-removal is potentially not a huge deal, and even many married physicians needn't worry, especially if you can "lower" your income or switch back (see below).

Loan payments are calculated based on your "adjusted" gross income, which takes some deductions into account. If your income jumps, you can "reduce" it by contributing to pretax accounts, such as your (non-Roth) 401(k)/403(b), 457(b), or HSA plans. Most academic jobs have both a 403(b) and 457(b), each with a $19,000 contribution limit. A few clicks and you can erase $38,000 in income from your taxes (and reduce next year's payments by $3,800). We'll talk about this in detail in the Maximizing PSLF chapter.

THE SWITCHBACK LOOPHOLE

The choice to enter REPAYE is not binding. In trying to close several loopholes, the feds left one open: as long as you still have a partial financial hardship, you can still switch back from REPAYE to IBR or PAYE. So, if it looks like your uncapped 10% payment is finally going to be too big, you can go back down to your "lower" capped 15% IBR (or 10% PAYE payments) while you still qualify. Likewise, if your spouse is going back to work or destined for a huge raise, you could switch back and file separately to avoid having your income considered together.

In both cases, you have to anticipate these changes and make the switch before your salary/salaries is/are so high that you no longer qualify, but this would still allow you the training years of lower payments and subsidized interest.

The main downside of switching plans is the capitalization of accrued interest. When transferring out of IBR, you must also make either 1) a big "standard" repayment and have the month counts towards PSLF or 2) a reduced payment ($5), but the month won't count, and you'll be delaying filing for PSLF by a month.

There is sometimes a 1-month administrative hold when switching in and out of REPAYE and PAYE, particularly if you do so near the annual certification deadline (thus also potentially causing a 1-month delay in PSLF).

We'll discuss this again in greater detail in a minute.

FOR WHOM THIS GENERALLY MATTERS:

Other than new graduates making their first election, there are a few groups of people who should look into switching.

GROUP 1: PEOPLE IN IBR WHO WANT PSLF

All of this is most relevant for people trying to minimize monthly payments for eventual forgiveness under the Public Service Loan Forgiveness program. The goal for income-driven repayment and PSLF is to pay the absolute minimum possible per month for 120 payments (10 years) in order to maximize the currently unlimited (but mostly untested) tax-free loan forgiveness.

This plan starts in residency when income is low, continues throughout training (the longer the better), and ends up with as few years as possible at the higher-earning attending level to eat away at your potential forgiveness. Spousal income aside, 10% AGI payments under REPAYE will be lower than 15% payments in IBR. The downside to switching is interest capitalization, but not only is this usually mitigated by the interest subsidy, it's actually irrelevant if your loans are forgiven (consider the subsidy in this case to be hedging your bets against PSLF). Residents in IBR should instead mostly be residents in REPAYE (the exceptions being if you were relying on the married-filing-separately loophole to exclude your spouse's income or if you already make a cap-busting amount of money).

GROUP 2: PEOPLE WHO CAN'T AFFORD IBR PAYMENTS

People forbearing because they can't afford IBR payments and don't qualify for PAYE could instead enter REPAYE in order to lower their monthly payments by a third and start making some payments. This is a big benefit versus forbearance because of the half unpaid interest subsidy, which really slows down interest accumulation. The caveat here is that if you couldn't afford IBR, you still might not be able to afford REPAYE. If 10% is still not affordable, then you should see what kind of rate you get from private refinancing, as a couple companies have plans for residents that require between $75-$100/month during training and generally offer lower interest rates. Forbeared loans don't have any of the IDR benefits, and they grow fast.

GROUP 3: PEOPLE IN PAYE WHO ARE CURRENTLY ACCRUING A LOT OF INTEREST

While your monthly payments won't change, the amount of unpaid interest accumulating will be cut in half. This is meaningless if you are going for PSLF since the total amount of your forgiven loan doesn't matter to you (only the amount you spent to get there). Outside of PSLF, this could be a big deal, particularly if you have a fair amount of residency left. See take-home points below.

A WORD ON NON-PSLF LONG-TERM FORGIVENESS

Basically no one should really be going for the 20/25-year forgiveness unless you went to private college and med school, racked up an incredible amount of debt, but then went on to earn peanuts for a non-PSLF eligible job. But if that describes your plan, PAYE is 20 years. REPAYE is 25 years (just like IBR) if you have graduate loans (which you do). So, definitely worth switching from IBR to REPAYE. The choice if currently in PAYE is more complicated (see next chapter). Unlike PSLF, this forgiven amount is taxed as income for all income-driven repayment plans (the more you get forgiven, the more you owe the IRS as a big tax bomb).

Ick. If you're not minimizing payments to get the most out of PSLF, you should instead be maximizing them to get rid of this high-interest debt.

TAKE-HOME POINTS

REPAYE is a big deal with two big draws: Compared with IBR, it has lower monthly payments. Compared with both IBR and PAYE, there's the new unpaid interest subsidy. Some "loopholes" are closed (no married filing separately loophole and no monthly payment cap), but these may not be relevant to your situation. Residents need to consider REPAYE seriously.

There is no true "average" medical student, because even people who carry an average amount of debt may have different circumstances. That said, for the average unmarried resident, REPAYE during residency is likely to be the best choice, followed by (staying in) PAYE.

FOR IBR:

- If you're doing IBR, you owe it to yourself to run some numbers to see if REPAYE is for you. The main immediate downside will be interest capitalization and potentially losing one month of PSLF-qualifying payment during the switch. Is that loss a big deal? Well, how much is your standard monthly payment? That average $50k earning resident saves $130 bucks a month in REPAYE over IBR. That's $1,560 a year. For example, the standard payment for a $200k loan is $2,302. In this case, it would take over a year to break even on the long-term costs PSLF-wise despite the immediate payment reduction.

- The main long-term downside could be if your future salary breaks through the cap. As above, this may not be a realistic problem for you, and even if it is, will likely take some time to undo the money you saved. You may also be able to preempt this by switching back to IBR while you still qualify.

FOR PAYE

- If you're doing PAYE, you won't save any money on your monthly payment, but if you have a high debt/income ratio (and many of you do), then you can potentially save a lot of money due to the new unpaid interest subsidy. If you're married, this will depend on your spouse's income and debt burden as well.

- If you're already in PAYE and set on PSLF, there is no significant reason to switch, because you won't benefit from the interest subsidy (it was all going to be forgiven anyway). If the government makes you uneasy, REPAYE can help you hedge your bets by lowering your effective interest rate while in training.

- If you're definitely not going for PSLF, then there is no harm in applying to the resident-friendly private companies to see what the industry can offer you. If the rates they offer are lower than your effective REPAYE rate, then consider refinancing. Alternatively, if you need the even lower payments ($75 or $100/month) those banks offer in order to not enter forbearance, then refinance. If you're scared about the future and want to lock in a relatively lower interest rate now instead of temporarily using REPAYE, then refinance (this would be a gut move, not a logical one).

- If you're not sure about doing PSLF and are still experiencing negative amortization, then consider switching to REPAYE: this will keep your qualifying payments at the lowest possible amount while also limiting the growth of painfully accruing interest: a healthy middle ground.

EXTRA MONEY AND REPAYE

One big question that comes up frequently is if it's possible to pay extra money on top of the calculated REPAYE monthly amount and still qualify for the interest subsidy. The answer is yes, but it might not be worth it.

Emphasis mine:

> *"Under the REPAYE Plan, if* **your calculated monthly payment** *doesn't cover all of the interest that accrues, the government will pay*
>
> - *all of the remaining interest that is due on your subsidized loans (including the subsidized portion of a consolidation loan) for up to three consecutive years from the date you begin repaying your loans under the REPAYE Plan, and half of the remaining interest on your subsidized loans following this three-year period; and*
>
> - *half of the remaining interest that is due on your unsubsidized loans (including the unsubsidized portion of a consolidation loan), during all periods."*

So yes, if you're doing REPAYE to get that sweet interest subsidy and wanted to pay down your loans faster, you can. Technically, the subsidy is based on what REPAYE says you need to be paying every month, not on what you actually choose to pay.

Many have also questioned if you need to "time" the interest subsidy (i.e. make the second payment immediately after the subsidy is applied before more unpaid interest accrues in order to not reduce the amount of unpaid interest and thus decrease the subsidy). Based on the language of the policy, this is not the case. Furthermore, not all servicers apply the subsidy in the same way and many do not make it clear exactly when or how this occurs. If you want to be extra cautious and time your payments, you're probably going to need to make a phone call. And when you make a phone call, be prepared to receive incorrect information.

However, unless you can pay enough extra to dent the principal, there isn't much point. Remember that interest in REPAYE doesn't capitalize and that you can't directly pay down the principal until all the accrued interest has been taken care of. Chipping away a few extra bucks of interest here and there isn't going to change the rate of interesting accrual (just the total amount that's sitting there). As a result, in this situation, it makes sense to put this money somewhere else, even just an interest-bearing savings account. The interest you earn on the saved up money would then help mitigate the interest on your loans. Make your money work for you.

FURTHER FACETS OF INCOME-DRIVEN REPAYMENT

UNDERGRADUATE OR OLD GRAD SCHOOL LOANS DURING MEDICAL SCHOOL

While you can't enter repayment for the loans you've borrowed for your current schooling due to their "in-school" status, you *can* decline the normal in-school deferment on your old loans. You can even do a federal consolidation early so you can pick your servicer (especially helpful if you have more than one) and streamline your loan statements. After graduating, you can simply file for a consolidation add-on to add your med school loans to the consolidation.

Most medical students without significantly employed spouses would qualify for $0 payments under IDR plans. If you have unsubsidized loans from undergrad that would be accruing interest during school, it makes sense to decline the in-school deferment and put those loans into the REPAYE program. Due to the unpaid interest subsidy, you'd cut the effective interest rate in half and save a bunch of money.

A relevant bit from the official PSLF Q&A:

1. *If I return to school and qualify for an in-school deferment on my Direct Loans that are in repayment, can I decline the deferment and make qualifying PSLF payments while I'm in school?*

   Yes. You may decline an in-school deferment on your loans that are in repayment status and make qualifying payments on those loans while you are in school. Remember, in order for your payments to qualify for PSLF, you must be employed full-time by a public service organization while you attend school. Note: If you receive new Direct Subsidized Loans or Direct Unsubsidized Loans when you return to school, you will not be able to make qualifying PSLF payments on those loans while you are in school. Any new Direct Subsidized Loans or Direct Unsubsidized Loans you receive will not enter repayment until the end of the six-month grace period. Although you could voluntarily make payments on your new Direct Subsidized Loans and Direct Unsubsidized Loans while you are in school or during your grace period, those payments would not count toward PSLF.

So those $0 payments won't work for achieving PSLF (unless you were somehow also working full-time for a qualifying non-profit), but they would count toward the baked-in IDR forgiveness that you should probably be ignoring. Most important would be the interest subsidy, but this makes sense only for unsubsidized loans. Subsidized loans don't accrue interest while in school, so if all of you have from your prior education are subsidized loans, there isn't much to be gained as there isn't any accruing interest to be unpaid and subsequently subsidized.

SWITCHING FROM REPAYE

There has been a lot of confusion from borrowers concerning whether or not REPAYE, with its partial interest subsidy, is a good choice for people with high future income (e.g. residents). The main concern is what happens after training when salaries increase and the possibility of breaking past the monthly payment cap, which could make you lose money (in the context of trying to minimize payments in anticipation of PSLF).

Brief aside: If you're just trying to pay off your loans in an efficient way, breaking past the cap should be mostly irrelevant–you should be trying to pay down your loans as fast as possible anyway.

So, if you call your federal loan servicer but don't ask the right questions, your servicer may lead you astray in how they answer questions about the terms of the REPAYE program. It's misleading but technically true: if you are making so much money that you break past the REPAYE cap, you absolutely cannot switch back to PAYE or IBR.

That's **not** because you aren't allowed to switch out of REPAYE in general (you are), but because at that point you would no longer have a "partial financial hardship" and thus no longer qualify for those plans to begin with. Your servicer is able to provide information and advice but don't for a second think that they don't have a vested *interest* in your payments (see what I did there?). A simple rule of thumb is that if you owe more on your loans than you make in a year, you definitely still qualify for your income-driven repayment plan.

Remember that what is actually used for payment calculations is not your gross income but your discretionary income: your gross income minus 150% of the federal poverty line for your family size. The official rule is that if your calculated monthly PAYE/IBR payment (whichever you qualify for) using 10/15% of your discretionary income is less than the standard 10-year repayment, then you still qualify. Put differently, if you put your income into the federal calculator and it spits out an IDR payment lower than the standard, then your income qualifies for you that IDR plan.

As we discussed break-even points earlier, once you hit your break-even salary you have no unpaid interest and thus no REPAYE interest subsidy. For a $200,000 loan at 6%, that's a salary of about $138,000. At this point, REPAYE isn't offering you anything over PAYE.

There is a simple solution for forward-thinking borrowers who want to take advantage of the REPAYE benefits but don't want to tie themselves to higher future payments: switch back before you make good money.

You can switch from REPAYE to PAYE as long as you still qualify for PAYE. If you didn't qualify for PAYE to begin with due to older loans, then you can switch back to IBR instead. Do this at the end of your training and the problem is solved. (Technically, many people could do it even once out in practice; it all depends on how much you borrowed versus how much you/your family makes per year. You can use the calculator to see what household income you'll need to break past the threshold.) An endocrinologist who borrowed $200k but makes $150k annually would qualify forever.

Also note that since most people generally use tax returns and not pay stubs to verify income, there is generally a delay between when your income rises and when your taxes reflect that increase. This isn't the way servicers would like it, but it's the reality on the ground. You could be an attending as of July 2017, but when you resubmit income verification in the fall of 2017 for REPAYE, you'll be submitting your 2016 tax return, which was a combination of your last two PGY years of training. The annual certification does indeed ask you if your current income has changed from your taxes. In order to answer this question truthfully and avoid the possibility of getting stumped by a paystub request, one would just certify your income early before starting your new job. Because most MD jobs start in July, it's generally a good thing to have your annual certification take place in June before your income increases for the year, something we will discuss in the chapter on Direct Consolidation.

The bottom line is that you absolutely can switch out of REPAYE—you just have to be a little bit thoughtful on when you want to switch out to not miss the window. REPAYE makes the most sense for many if not most residents. For people who aren't going for PSLF (especially if they've borrowed smaller amounts and won't enjoy a big interest subsidy), no-cost private refinancing may be a better choice.

The briefest verbiage for this plan-switch information comes from the plan breakdown table for official IDR Plans Q&A (emphasis mine):

> *Leaving the Plan (REPAYE)*
>
> *If you choose to leave this plan, you may change to any other repayment plan* **for which you are eligible**

If you talk to your servicer and they say otherwise, ask them to explain exactly why and get to the bottom of it. Because they are wrong.

SWITCHING OUT OF IBR

Switching out of PAYE or REPAYE is straightforward. You may be placed on a 1-month administrative forbearance while the servicer makes the change (especially if you submit your annual certification toward the deadline), but otherwise the process should be smooth and automatic.

However, to switch out of IBR, this annoying thing happens:

> *If you leave this plan, you will be placed on the Standard Repayment Plan. If you want to change to a different repayment plan, you must first make at least one payment under the Standard Repayment Plan, or one payment under a reduced payment forbearance (you may request a reduced-payment forbearance if you can't afford the Standard Repayment Plan payment).*

This was presumably done to stop people from immediately jumping ship from IBR to PAYE. In practice, the "reduced-payment" requirement is $5. So, you don't *need* to shell over a few thousand to cover a month's standard repayment. On the other hand, a reduced-payment month won't count towards PSLF.

Additionally, switching plans will cause all of your accrued interest to capitalize. If you've been out for a few years making the typical negative amortizing IBR payments during residency, you may have a sizable chunk of accumulated interest sitting around.

An illustrative example:

- $200k loan @ 6.8% accrues $13.6k per year

- Assuming a $50k salary and $400/month IBR payment, the annual unpaid interest is $8,800

- After 2 years of residency, that's $17.6k accrued interest. After 3 years, it's $26.4k.

- Switching from IBR to PAYE after two or three years results in a new loan balance of $217.6k and $226.4k respectively. From that point on, the annual interest then would increase to $14.7k and $15.4k.

In this example, your monthly payment is reduced from $400 in IBR to around $266 under PAYE or REPAYE, which is great from a cash flow perspective and for PSLF. But now your loans may be growing faster than ever (both from the capitalized interest on top of the fact that you are simply paying less of it).

By cutting those payments down from 15% to 10%, you'll be taking an even bigger hit in terms of your loan growth, unless you switch to REPAYE and are getting a nice subsidy. Keep in mind however that the interest that accrued while you were in school capitalized when you graduated, so you don't have a ton to worry about if you're fresh out of school or relatively close.

Switching to REPAYE for the interest subsidy is one thing, but outside of desperate cash flow needs, the main reason to switch from IBR to PAYE is really only to double down for PSLF. In order to maximize the gains of public service loan forgiveness, you want to spend the least amount possible during your 120 qualifying payments. The spiraling balance is then irrelevant because it's going to be forgiven. When deciding if switching makes sense, don't forget you'll need to make one more big attending or "standard" payment if you switch while in training and lose a smaller residency-sized payment (losing up to $2,300 on the above example and basically washing 17 months of that reduced monthly payment away). You may decide that the lower payments now are worth it regardless, which they basically will be unless you're within your final two years of training. PAYE vs REPAYE

If you've gotten this far, you know that PAYE and REPAYE have a lot in common. But there are differences that can make one or the other the better choice.

INTEREST CAPITALIZATION CAP VS INTEREST SUBSIDY

To start, what about that PAYE interest capitalization cap? How does that compare to the REPAYE interest subsidy?

Poorly! There are reasons PAYE can be a better choice for many borrowers, but the interest capitalization cap isn't really one of them.

As you may recall, within the PAYE plan, any accrued interest that capitalizes is limited to 10% of the original principal amount when you enter repayment. What this means is that no matter how much interest accrues, the maximum principal amount after capitalization at any point is the original amount + 10%. Which means that over the long term, the *rate* of interest accrual is capped (but not the amount, of course). When does interest capitalize within the PAYE program? When you lose your partial financial hardship, which often happens at some point during attendinghood depending on how much you owe vs. how much you make.

An example would be if you had a $200k loan with $50k in accrued interest; after capitalization in PAYE, the loan would be $220k with $30k in accrued interest instead of $250k, which means at 6.8%, $14,960 accrues per year instead of $17,000. This may or may not be a big deal.

In contrast, REPAYE has a subsidy that pays half of the unpaid accrued interest on a monthly basis. But the real reason the cap itself is never better than the subsidy is because REPAYE interest **never capitalizes** unless you leave the plan. Because there is no hardship requirement, your interest will continue to accrue at the same rate it always has. Only if you try to change back to a different repayment plan (say, to lower payments as a high-earning attending using the married-filing-separately loophole) would your interest capitalize. That $200k loan in REPAYE will always accrue the same amount of interest every year (until you begin to pay down the principal, of course).

SO, WHEN DOES PAYE BEAT REPAYE THEN?

For single people or married people filing jointly, PAYE and REPAYE payments will always be the same (10% of AGI) until income rises high enough such that 10% of your income is greater than the 10-year standard payment calculated based on your original loan amount when you enter repayment. At this point, PAYE caps at that amount while REPAYE continues to grow with growing income. Big money means bigger payments. This is actually good from the perspective of minimizing the amount of interest that accrues while paying your loan off and thus saving money overall but bad from the perspective of minimizing payments for possible loan forgiveness or to fund your high-rolling lifestyle.

The other big difference is when you rely on filing taxes separately from your spouse in order to get low payments with PAYE, a trick/loophole closed by REPAYE.

So, PAYE will frequently "beat" REPAYE in three scenarios:

1. A spouse earns a significant income without holding significant federal student loans.

2. When your adjusted gross income rises beyond the standard "cap." For a $200k loan at 6.8% for example, that amount is around $295,000 a year for a single filer.

3. If your income to loan ratio means you're not getting an interest subsidy. In this case, your payments are capped at standard and you're free to use the loopholes you need.

You can run these scenarios easily in one of the calculators listed at the end of the book (just put different salaries and look at the first monthly payment). When either of these situations is about to happen while in REPAYE, it's permissible to switch to PAYE (if eligible) or IBR (if that still works out in your favor). Note that switching to PAYE/IBR to avoid the spousal income issue requires that you file taxes separately and then submit your IDR income certification paperwork, so you can't simply do this right before you start a new job without some planning. You typically file your taxes by April, but most people certify in the summer or fall.

Bottom line: the likelihood of PAYE being better than REPAYE in the future isn't necessarily a reason to avoid REPAYE in the present if it otherwise makes sense.

WHAT ABOUT OVER THE SUPER LONG TERM, LIKE 20 VS 25-YEAR FORGIVENESS?

Ah, yes, the super long-term baked-in forgiveness that sounds perfect for someone with $500k in student loans who wants to work part-time making $150k forever. See the chapter on Long-Term Loan Forgiveness.

FEDERAL "DIRECT" CONSOLIDATION

When you get federal student loans from the government for medical school, you don't just get one loan: you get at least one per year. Back in the day when graduate students still received subsidized loans, many borrowers would receive three: one subsidized, one unsubsidized, and often a small subsidized "low-interest" (5%) Perkins loan. Now, in practice, holding on to multiple loans doesn't really affect your daily life much. Your federal loan servicer (the company that takes your payments) will apply your payments automatically across all of your DIRECT loans for you (your Perkins loans, if you have any, will be due separately from the rest). After setting up auto debit for your loans, the monthly payments are withdrawn and applied appropriately automatically. You'll even get a small rate discount. It's a set-it and forget-it situation.

Consolidating your federal loans into a federal Direct Consolidation from the federal government (as opposed to private refinancing/consolidation, discussed in detail later) does make things look nice and tidy in that you'll now have a single loan with a weighted-average interest rate based on the rates of the individual loans it replaced, but this paperwork trick isn't particularly meaningful in and of itself. Unlike private refinance options, you're guaranteed to not save a single dime on the interest rate. In fact, a slight rounding change could give you a trivially higher rate: the new loan's rate is rounded up to the nearest one-eighth of 1%. The subsidized loans within a consolidation maintain their subsidized status, though any Perkins loans do not.

But there are definitely a few reasons why you should consolidate your loans, particularly as early as you can after graduation, in large part due to the REPAYE program. And there's a double reason if you're considering PSLF.

In short, starting your federal consolidation when you finish medical school will do three things to save you money:

1. Reduce the amount of capitalized interest on your loan, which reduces the rate at which it will grow for a long time

2. Temporarily increase the amount of your REPAYE unpaid-interest subsidy

3. Help you achieve loan forgiveness a few months faster

4. Max out the student loan interest deduction for the year of graduation

We'll discuss each of these in detail followed by brief step by step instructions. Stay with me.

CONSOLIDATING TO MAKE YOUR LOANS IDR & PSLF ELIGIBLE

The first benefit of Direct consolidation is that it can make more of your debt eligible for income-driven repayment (IDR) and public service loan forgiveness (PSLF). Not all loans you can get for financial aid are eligible for PSLF, only Direct loans are: Direct loans are those provided "directly" by the federal government: Direct Stafford (for older borrowers), Direct Subsidized (for undergrads only), Direct Unsubsidized (the most common med school loan), Direct PLUS (higher interest rate for big borrowers), and Direct Consolidation.

If you want to have your Perkins loans forgiven, then consolidation is the only way. Perkins loans are normally automatically put on their own separate 10-year repayment, so consolidation is also the only way to have Perkins loans included within an income-driven repayment plan, which would reduce the amount you pay monthly if you're worried about cash flow problems (note: you can't forbear a Perkins loan). Most medical students don't get a ton in Perkins a year, so we're not talking about huge amounts of money (and now that the Perkins program was canceled in September 2017, no one will be getting any new Perkins loans at all). That being said, having my $4,500 in Perkins forgiven would be another $4,500+ that I didn't have to pay and $50/month less in payments.

IMPORTANT CAVEAT:

If you've already been repaying your loans and are wondering if you should consolidate in order to add your Perkins: Achieving loan forgiveness through the PSLF program is based on making 120 qualifying monthly payments on a given loan. When you consolidate, the feds pay off your old loans and create a new consolidation loan in their place. Because the consolidation is a new loan, the monthly payment count resets to zero. Any payments you've made towards your loans prior to this do not count toward the PSLF required 120.

CONSOLIDATING AT THE END OF SCHOOL SAVES YOU MONEY

The key facet to saving money with federal consolidation is that consolidation loans have no grace period. Normally, you have a mandatory 6-month grace period starting at the end of graduation before you begin paying back any money. If you graduate at the beginning of May, you normally won't be paying anything until November. During this grace period, interest continues to accrue and is then capitalized (added to the principal) at the end when you enter repayment. And, of course, you also won't start making any payments toward PSLF until 6 months after graduation either.

The only way to waive the grace period is to consolidate:

> *If you want to immediately begin making qualifying payments on your federal student loans as soon as you leave school, you may consolidate your loans into a Direct Consolidation Loan during your grace period and enter repayment right away.*

For the following example, let's assume you file for consolidation at the end of school in May, which is then processed in June. You'll probably lose one or two months out of the 6-month grace period to the consolidation process. Another 4 weeks later to set up re-payment, and your first payment might start in July, which coinci-dentally is when you start working. The example numbers here are based on a $200,000 loan at 6% with an intern salary of $50k and a household size of 1 (some reasonable numbers for purely illustrative purposes; as always, do your own math).

1. Less capitalized interest. The interest accrued during school will capitalize when you consolidate instead of after an addi-tional six months of accrued interest. With $200k @ 6%, that's $6,000 of interest that won't be part of the principal accruing its own interest. That change in capitalization would result in around $360/year less interest accruing at the above rate. Note: If your loans are eventually forgiven as part of PSLF, this part would be irrelevant.

2. The REPAYE interest subsidy kicks in earlier. This assumes, of course, that you don't already have low-debt/high-income mis-match and will be receiving one in the first place. In our above example with a solo $50k intern salary, the projected monthly payment is about $270/month. $1,000 of interest accrues per month on the $200,000 loan. $730 of that is unpaid, and thus $365 is forgiven. Every month. An extra four months in REPAYE could save you $1,460 (again, I'm assuming you'll lose a couple of months in the consolidation/repayment process). This part also won't matter if you eventually achieve PSLF.

But it's actually better than that example: you typically certify your application for income-driven repayment plans using last year's tax filings. The tax year prior was half of your MS3 and MS4 years, when you probably had little to no taxable income, which would result in a $0 monthly payment: $500 would be forgiven each month ($2,000 over 4 months) while making $3,240 ($270 x 12) less in payments during your intern year. Now that is real savings even if you do PSLF.

A few years ago, some of the servicers wised up to the $0/month trick that people were commonly using when they filed for IDR at the end of grace period, and they sometimes asked for pay stubs from your intern year (the application also started asking if your income had "changed significantly" since your prior tax return), which meant that people who wanted a $0 qualifying IDR payment had to start fibbing and hope theirs was one of the servicers that didn't always ask for proof.

We're in a better place now because the application has changed again to specifically ask about any income decreases (not changes), but by consolidating early and applying for your repayment plan before you start your intern year, you *actually don't have any new income to report regardless*, your circumstances haven't changed since last year, and a $0 reported income is kosher again. By the federal government's own rules (see IDR FAQ #46), you don't have to update the servicers with new income numbers if your income changes before the annual income recertification, so once you have $0/month payments for the year, you're safe until the following year.

Yes, this means that—unless you have spousal income to account for—every intern can qualify for a REPAYE interest subsidy: $0 payments mean you'll always have unpaid interest. Even those planning on private refinancing will likely want to wait until they've enjoyed the fruits of the subsidy for a year.

Having $0 payments is essentially forbearing your intern year without any of the downsides and all of the upsides of making regularly scheduled income-based payments (no interest capitalization, qualified towards PSLF and long-term loan forgiveness, interest subsidy in REPAYE, etc.).

3. Earlier qualifying PSLF payments. Waiving the six-month grace period means a few more months of making payments as a low-income resident and a few months less as a high-earning attending. As an example, the standard 10-year repayment on that $200k loan is $,2302/month. If you were able to start repayment in July instead of November, those 4 months at $0 instead of $2,302 could save you $9,208 when it comes time to file for PSLF.

4. If you have low or $0 payments, you'd think that you would pay little to no interest and thus get no deduction on your taxes. However, long story short, the consolidation loan "pays" off all of the interest on your loans that accrued while you were in school, to the tune of likely far more than the $2,500 maximum deduction.

Note: The government specifically states that $0/month payments count toward PSLF **when that is the calculated payment under a qualifying repayment plan** (see PSLF FAQ #24). If you consolidate in a timely fashion after graduation, such a payment will be the result of a calculation based on the honest truth and completely in keeping with everything official out there.

HOW TO CONSOLIDATE

STEP 1:

File taxes on time in April of your fourth/final year of medical school (or at least before you graduate). You can do this for free in multiple ways online. File even if you didn't make money; it'll make things easier, as it will document your (lack of) income and will only take a few minutes. You won't have pay stubs yet, so your tax return is all you have.

STEP 2:

Your loans must be out of "in-school" status (e.g. graduated or grace period) to file for consolidation. So, once you graduate, immediately file for a federal loan consolidation by visiting studentloans.gov. Note: do not fill in the box with your "grace period end date" as this will delay the consolidation from taking place until the end of your grace period (i.e. item 17 on the paper application found at https://static.studentloans.gov/images/ApplicationAndPromissoryNote.pdf), which is exactly what we're trying to avoid. More information about which loans are federal consolidation-eligible is available at https://studentaid.ed.gov/sa/repay-loans/consolidation in case you have some rare ones not in the Loan Eligibility table in the Federal Repayment Options chapter. Note that you can see all of your loans listed, their total amounts (principal and interest), and your "enrollment status" (to confirm that the feds know you've graduated) using NSLDS (https://www.nslds.ed.gov).

You get to pick your servicer as part of your application. If you're considering PSLF at all, you may as well pick FedLoan, as you'll be transferred to them whenever you submit your first PSLF employment certification form anyway. If not, it would be hard to know which to pick from the four consolidation choices: Nelnet, FedLoan, Great Lakes, and Navient. The feds actually periodically release student loan data, including an overall borrower satisfaction survey, with recent values ranging from around 60 to 70%. Great Lakes was consistently the "best" from this small spread. Navient is the most hated. If you're sure you don't want PSLF, I'd pick Great Lakes.

At the same time as your consolidation, you'll also be applying for the IDR plan you want to use to pay off your new consolidation loan, which will likely be REPAYE.

STEP 3:

Ideally, after two months or so you'll be the proud owner of a lot of debt in one place and a payment plan to start taking care of it. Once your servicer lets you know that you've entered repayment, make sure to sign up for their auto-debit program to make payments automatically through your checking account if available: auto-debit gets you an additional 0.25% interest rate reduction. If your payments are $0, they probably won't give you the option or won't apply the discount, but if you can, definitely do it. If you have non-zero payments, you'll get the reduction. In our example above, the auto-pay reduction saves you an extra $500.

Things may go wrong, so follow up if things don't start moving after 6 weeks. If you have multiple loans from multiple schools with multiple servicers, you may run into more problems. Note that it's also possible that your school and servicers may temporarily forget to update your loan status from "in-school" (not consolidation eligible) to "graduated" or "grace period" (consolidation eligible), so check on NSLDS and call your school and servicers if things don't progress after graduation.

UNDERGRADUATE LOANS

If you have undergrad loans, you could consolidate those at any point during med school and then file a "Direct Consolidation Loan Request to Add Loans" for the med school loans after graduation. I'm honestly not sure how much if any time that will save you, but it could potentially help prevent some of the difficulties associated with your servicer finding and paying off a bunch of different loans in a timely manner.

As we discussed in the "Further Facets of Income-Driven Repayment" chapter, you might save some money on interest by consolidating old undergraduate unsubsidized loans, waiving the in-school deferment, and entering REPAYE for those loans to get the interest subsidy. But outside of that situation, I'd personally just go with the one-step method after graduation.

$0 PAYMENTS

It's important to realize that zero-dollar payments will temporarily result in more disposable income than you may otherwise have in the future. The typical annual increase in your residency salary will make up some of the difference when you actually start making payments, but if you are living paycheck to paycheck as an intern with $0 payments, you need to consider how you will handle your loan payments in the subsequent years when your payments increase to reflect your actual income.

PARTING THOUGHTS ON CONSOLIDATION

None of this deal-breaking stuff. If you're already in repayment and haven't done this, don't kick yourself. You'll note that getting PSLF negates some of the extra plusses while not doing PSLF nullifies others. Early consolidation is a fantastic return on a small investment of time, but the fact that you're thinking about your debt and seriously want to take care of it is more important than the money you'll save.

So, in the end, the take-home points:

- Most of the loans that can be forgiven are automatically PSLF eligible.

- Perkins loans are the exception, which if you have them are typically a small fraction of your total debt. Adding them to a Direct Consolidation will make them eligible.

- Consolidating your loans immediately after graduating medical school can allow you to enter repayment immediately at the start of residency by foregoing/erasing the traditional mandatory six-month grace period, which can save you money by reducing interest capitalization, increasing your REPAYE subsidy, allowing for $0/month payments, and helping you reach loan forgiveness (if applicable) with fewer attending-sized payments.

- If you owe so little that the REPAYE subsidy is nominal and your effective interest rate is still high, you may consider private refinance to reduce your interest rate when appropriate.

THE PAIN OF FORBEARANCE

PENNY WISE, POUND FOOLISH.

People often chase sales and discounts on basically piddling amounts of money while letting their loans fester at high rates for inappropriate lengths of time. It's silly to clip coupons and then ignore your loans. While your life circumstances may ultimately force your hand, forbearance is probably the worst financial decision you can make during residency.

CAPITALIZED LOAN AMOUNTS AT 6% AFTER YEARS OF FORBEARANCE

LOAN AMOUNT	1	2	3	4	5
$100,000	$106,000	$112,000	$118,000	$124,000	$130,000
$150,000	$159,000	$168,000	$177,000	$186,000	$195,000
$200,000	$212,000	$224,000	$236,000	$248,000	$260,000
$250,000	$265,000	$280,000	$295,000	$310,000	$325,000
$300,000	$318,000	$336,000	$354,000	$372,000	$390,000
$350,000	$371,000	$392,000	$413,000	$434,000	$455,000
$400,000	$424,000	$448,000	$472,000	$496,000	$520,000
$450,000	$477,000	$504,000	$531,000	$558,000	$585,000
$500,000	$530,000	$560,000	$590,000	$620,000	$650,000

THE GOOD OF FORBEARANCE:

You get to temporarily not make payments on your loans, at least for the duration of your training.

THE BAD OF FORBEARANCE:

Interest continues to accumulate on all loans (subsidies and unsubsidized). You get no IDR-derived interest subsidy and you get no autopay rate reduction. Then, at the end of the forbearance period, the interest capitalizes. In other words, the longer you forbear, the worse things get. PSLF for doctors is a much better deal when you take the low payments of residency into account, so forbearance can ruin that too:

Making three extra years of standard repayment-sized payments (due to a forbearance) in order to achieve PSLF on a $200,000 loan could result in spending an extra **$80,000**.

YOU USUALLY DON'T NEED TO FORBEAR

What many people don't realize is that you don't need to forbear your loans when you don't make any money; you usually just need to recertify your income to reduce your income-driven repayment. If you are currently earning zero dollars a month, then your income-based payment will be zero dollars a month. That is substantially better than forbearing because you're then still eligible for the benefits of an IDR plan: For example, you'll still get half the accrued interest forgiveness part of the REPAYE plan. When you start making money again, the interest that has accrued will not capitalize onto the principal, because you were not forbearing. You were simply making smaller (zero dollar) payments. When it comes to recertifying your income, you should consider recertifying if your income drops (e.g. if a spouse stops working or gets a pay cut, because your residency salary is unlikely to change meaningfully unless you are on medical leave). However, if your income rises, you should wait until you receive the annual demand to do so, because recertifying early will simply raise your payments earlier.

Scenario: you and your spouse are both fully employed and diligently paying off your student loans to the extent you can. One of you gets pregnant and decides to take a year off from work to raise the baby. Money is now tighter, and your income-based payment is going to be a stretch. You consider forbearing. But you may not have to: your new lower calculated payment based on one income may be affordable.

Of course, it's possible that even a payment derived from only one income is too much to handle. So be it, life happens. Just be aware that forbearance should be your last option.

Needing to forbear as a resident is also a scenario where it's worth evaluating a no-cost private refinance. The monthly payments with a resident-friendly company during training are between $0-100, likely substantially less than your IDR payments. A worthwhile refinance will reduce your interest rate, and a 1% rate difference for a $200k loan is $2,000 per year.

DEFINITELY DON'T FORBEAR YOUR INTERN YEAR

As we discussed in the chapter on Direct Consolidation, many people should be able to swing $0 payments for intern year. This means that IDR costs no more than forbearance but has all the perks. So: forbearing unnecessarily during your intern year can easily cost thousands.

IDR INSTEAD

When you decide to enter IBR/PAYE/REPAYE instead of forbearance:

1. The government pays the unpaid interest on your subsidized loans for 3 years (if you have any). In REPAYE, the feds also waive half of the unpaid interest on your unsubsidized loans, effectively reducing your interest rate.

2. All monthly payments during residency count towards the 120 monthly payments (10 years) needed for public service loan

forgiveness. Even if you switch to forbearance later, the qualifying payments you make still count (they don't have to be consecutive). Since your remaining loan balance after 120 payments will be forgiven, it is in your best interest to have these payments be as small as possible, so don't waste your low-pay years as a resident unless you need to. This same logic applies to long-term IDR loan forgiveness as well.

THE COUNTERARGUMENT

Let's say you want to enter private practice and plan to make enough money that you just don't care about your loan amount (congrats to you for your high-paying specialty choice; just don't blow it all on your BMW and summer home). You just want to maximize your lifestyle during residency when money is tight and that $250-400 a month will make a big difference. Maybe you have kids to feed and/or daycares to pay for. That's fine too. It happens. If after considering all of your options, you simply can't afford to pay off your loans or have some private practice job lined up with a big student loan bonus, etc.—that's okay. At least you'll have a better idea of the pro/cons/consequences of the choice.

If the plan is to forbear, again, you should really consider IDR for a year (or two).

If forbearance is a sure thing, it's pretty unlikely you're bound for PSLF. In this case, it behooves you to look into private refinancing. While most companies don't offer plans that will work for a resident's depressing financial picture, there are a few that do, and—as we covered earlier—even relatively modest rate decreases can add up significantly over time. But before you do anything, make sure the money saved makes it worthwhile compared with staying with your federal loans (even while forbearing). It's a one-way street. If forgiveness is even a remote possibility, think long and hard before pulling the trigger.

DEFERMENT IS NOT FORBEARANCE

Some people use deferment and forbearance interchangeably, particularly older physicians who used to qualify for deferment during residency, but they're different. While both allow you "defer" making payments, the government pays the interest on any subsidized loans during a deferment (but not during forbearance).

This matters less now that graduate students don't receive subsidized loans anymore.

Residents used to meet criteria for the "economic hardship deferment" but no longer. Other deferments are the in-school deferment, military service, military post-active duty, unemployment, rehabilitation training, graduate fellowship, and the post-enrollment deferment (to automatically delay PLUS loans by 6-months, since they technically have no grace period).

KEEP IN MIND YOUR REALITY

The debt fact cards and most AAMC materials always compare strict-IDR versus forbearance followed by standard repayment, which minimizes the long-term benefit of making payments during residency by following it up with the extended (lazy) repayment term of IDR and its higher amount of interest payments. However, someone who is willing to put money down in residency is also someone who is likely to want to pay down his or her loans quickly. The bigger your salary, the higher your payment (until the cap in IBR/PAYE). If you were to stay in IDR but be aggressive and make additional payments as an attending, then you don't magically lose any of the money you save by using IDR as a resident: making interest payments, getting government money, and avoiding capitalization. The longer your residency, the greater this difference is. Don't be discouraged by looking at the official materials, the numbers are unlikely to reflect a proactive physician's capabilities.

In the end, how much you save by choosing IDR over forbearance depends on how much you borrowed and if PSLF is in your future.

For PSLF, every year of forbearance during training results in another year of attending size payments. For a $200k borrower, a 4-year forbearance could cost around $100,000 in extra payments.

For the DIY-er, the extra expenses can add up. The same $200k loan at 6% with a three-year residency/forbearance would result in extra unpaid interest of about $36k (including around $12k of which that could have been waived via REPAYE) followed by $2k/yr extra due to capitalized interest. The higher you will be paid as an attending relative to as a resident, the less meaningful the money saved and the more significant the money spent during residency.

Note, you can always make voluntary payments during a period of forbearance. Wanting to put money toward your loans does not preclude you from forbearing, and making a payment during forbearance does not obligate you to start making more payments.

FINAL THOUGHTS

The longer your residency/fellowship, the more money doing IDR with or without PSLF can save you and the more ridiculously your loans will balloon while in forbearance.

Forbearance is clearly the "wrong" choice financially and should be avoided if possible. But if making payments will crush you as a resident and you don't plan on working for a non-profit after training, then forbearance (or even private refinancing), at least during part of your training, could be the "right" choice for you.

But probably not.

PUBLIC SERVICE LOAN FORGIVENESS

PSLF is the holy grail of federal loan forgiveness. The master promissory note you signed when you took out your loans had this paragraph toward the end:

> *A Public Service Loan Forgiveness (PSLF) program is also available. Under this program, we will forgive the remaining balance due on your eligible Direct Loan Program loans after you have made 120 payments on those loans (after October 1, 2007) under certain repayment plans while you are employed full-time in certain public service jobs. The required 120 payments do not have to be consecutive. Qualifying repayment plans include the REPAYE Plan, the PAYE Plan, the IBR Plan, the ICR Plan, and the Standard Repayment Plan with a 10-year repayment period.*

That sums up the gist pretty nicely. So, achieving PSLF comes from the combination of a few critical components.

The PSLF formula:

Eligible Loans
+ Qualifying Payments
+ Qualifying Work
x 120 months (10 years)

= Public Service Loan Forgiveness

THE LOANS

PSLF is a government program run by the Department of Education for the forgiveness of government loans. Eligible loans are exclusively of the "Direct" variety: Stafford (older borrowers), subsidized, unsubsidized, PLUS, consolidation, etc. If you have other non-eligible federal loans (e.g. Perkins), you can often consolidate them into a DIRECT consolidation loan in order to be eligible.

Note that the 120 payments are calculated **per loan**, so if you consolidate, the counter resets. This means that you need to take care of any loan voodoo before you start making payments in order to not waste time/money. Again, go to www.nslds.ed.gov to find out what loans you have if you don't know. If the type of loan doesn't have the word "Direct" in it, it doesn't qualify for PSLF.

THE PAYMENTS

Payments must be on-time required monthly payments while in repayment while employed full-time. Extra payments, grace period payments, payments made during school, etc. do not count. It's 120 months, no shortcuts. As noted above, they do not have to be continuous payments. Also note that you must keep working full-time at the non-profit after you submit your forgiveness request until you actually receive forgiveness, which takes at least a few extra months to process.

In March 2018, a small provision in the "Consolidated Appropriations Act, 2018" set aside $350 million in additional funds to help out some unfortunate folks who were missing out on PSLF due to technicalities related to choosing a non-IDR plan for repayment for some/all of their 120 qualifying payments. The new program is being called the Temporary Expanded Public Service Loan Forgiveness (TEPSLF). In short, it makes the Graduated Repayment Plan, Extended Repayment Plan, Consolidation Standard Repayment Plan, and Consolidation Graduated Repayment Plan eligible for PSLF.

This money is available on a first-come, first-serve basis, and you apply after your initial PSLF application has been denied. You can learn more here: https://studentaid.ed.gov/sa/repay-loans/forgiveness-cancellation/public-service/temporary-expanded-public-service-loan-forgiveness

THE WORK

A qualifying public service job is defined as any full-time job at a government or non-profit, tax-exempt, 501(c)(3) organization. Most teaching hospitals fall under this category, and even some private hospitals fall under this designation. If you don't know, just ask. Better yet, search:

- http://501c3lookup.org/

- https://projects.propublica.org/nonprofits/ (you can even see the actual tax returns on ProPublica)

Keep in mind that many technically "nonprofit" hospitals do not directly employ physicians but rather contract with them. You have to be an actual employee of the institution as identified on your W2 to qualify. So that really luxurious "nonprofit" with the great salary in most cases isn't going to cut it. The general consensus is that being paid on a 1099 means you are an independent contractor (not an employee) and thus will not qualify. Hard to be directly employed by the non-profit if you're self-employed, right?

"Full-time" for purposes of PSLF is whatever is considered "full time" by your employer or 30 hours/week for at least 8 months/year, whichever is **more**.

Also note that up to three months of FMLA (Family Medical Leave Act) still count as full-time work for these purposes, so you won't necessarily delay PSLF by taking America's sorry excuse for maternity leave, taking care of family, or getting sick.

For each different eligible job contributing to the 120 months, you must submit a PSLF employment certification form. This is something you should do annually but absolutely at the minimum do at the end of your tenure at any facility. While you could theoretically go back and submit the form from your transitional internship 9 years later, doing it as you go would seem like a much safer bet. Once you submit your first employment certification form, your loan servicer will be switched to FedLoan (as opposed to one of the several others you may have been assigned to such as Nelnet, Navient, etc.), because FedLoan is the government's chosen servicer and thus the one handling government forgiveness. The more unusual your work circumstances, the more important it is to submit these forms every year.

These are the full eligibility criteria for PSLF-eligible employers:

- Government organizations at any level (federal, state, local, or tribal)

- Not-for-profit organizations that are tax-exempt under Section 501(c)(3) of the Internal Revenue Code

- Other types of not-for-profit organizations that provide certain types of "qualifying public services" and must not be a business organized for profit, a labor union, a partisan political organization, or an organization engaged in religious activities.

Qualifying public services include:

- Emergency management

- Military service

- Public safety

- Law enforcement

- Public interest law services

- Early childhood education (including licensed or regulated health care, Head Start, and State-funded pre-kindergarten)

- Public service for individuals with disabilities and the elderly

- Public health (including nurses, nurse practitioners, nurses in a clinical setting, and full-time professionals engaged in health care practitioner occupations and health care support occupations, as such terms are defined by the Bureau of Labor Statistics)

- Public education

- Public library services

- School library or other school-based services

So, it is the private nonprofits offering "qualifying" services that are the category at greatest risk for being denied. If your job isn't a 501(c)(3) but "should" qualify, submit your employment certification forms annually to prevent wasting your time and money planning for forgiveness that may forever remain out of reach. Even then, the Department of Education (which is now involved in a high-profile class-action lawsuit) has recently stated that FedLoan employment certifications for this third category "cannot be trusted" and may be denied. FedLoan has been known to accept some employment certification forms for 1099-earning independent contractors working at some non-profits, but there's no telling what's going to happen to those folks. A true 501(c)(3) or government job is by far the safer bet insofar as PSLF eligibility is concerned.

THE TAKEAWAY

PSLF isn't something you sign up for. It's something you automatically work toward when you make on-time monthly IDR payments. Similarly, the work verification also isn't a commitment to PSLF; it's just making sure your progress toward that possible goal is being counted appropriately so that you don't have any surprises or end up miscounting your qualifying months.

Keep in mind, there are several reasons to forget PSLF exists:

- You want to work in private practice.

- You plan to enter into a contract that will include loan forgiveness.

- You don't have a lot of debt (congrats).

- Your cynicism overpowers your hope that the program will continue to exist when you can reap its benefits (even the very first eligible folks didn't hit 120 payments until October 2017, and most of them were denied because they didn't read the fine print).

- You are set on forbearing during residency. As in, you are completely confident that the money you would need to pay for IDR during residency and fellowship will negatively impact your quality of life in such a way as to overcome the future financial benefit of having your loans forgiven (a tricky and likely shortsighted personal calculus).

But if you still want to:

- New graduates should consolidate their loans into a Direct Consolidation Loan as discussed previously.

- Sign up for an IDR plan: IBR, PAYE, or (most likely) REPAYE as soon as possible.

- Minimize payments by never paying more than you have to, which can include reducing your taxable income by maximizing tax deductions, contributing to pretax retirement accounts, etc. More about this in the next chapter.

- Fill out your employment certification forms annually (or at least when you change employers).

DOES PSLF MAKE SENSE FOR YOU?

TRAINING DURATION VS MONTHLY PAYE PAYMENTS AND TOTAL AMOUNT PAID TO ACHIEVE PSLF

	TRAINING DURATION IN YEARS						
PAYMENT YEAR (TAX YEAR)	3	4	5	6	7	8	9
1 (MS3/MS4)	$0	$0	$0	$0	$0	$0	$0
2 (MS4/PGY1)	$78	$78	$78	$78	$78	$78	$78
3 (PGY1/2)	$316	$316	$316	$316	$316	$316	$316
4 (PGY2/3)	$333	$333	$333	$333	$333	$333	$333
5 (PGY3/4)	$1,000	$349	$349	$349	$349	$349	$349
6 (PGY4/5)	$2,220	$1,000	$366	$366	$366	$366	$366
7 (PGY5/6)	$2,220	$2,220	$1,000	$383	$383	$383	$383
8 (PGY6/7)	$2,220	$2,220	$2,220	$1,000	$399	$399	$399
9 (PGY7/8)	$2,220	$2,220	$2,220	$2,220	$1,000	$416	$416
10 (PGY8/9)	$2,220	$2,220	$2,220	$2,220	$2,220	$1,000	$433
TOTAL PAID PRIOR TO PSLF	$154k	$131k	$109k	$87k	$65k	$43k	$37k

Assumptions: Consolidation after graduation with $0 payments during year 1 and half-intern-salary payments year 2. Intern salary is $55,000 increasing $2,000 a year per PGY year. Year transitioning between training and attending is an arbitrary mix (combined salary of ~$140,000) with a calculated monthly payment of $1,000. Attending salary every year caps at the standard 10-year monthly payment of $2,220. In reality, many people will not hit the salary cap, which requires a salary of about $280,000 in this example.

This chart illustrates a few important things:

1. While PSLF helps defray the cost of longer training, longer training won't be a good (financial) investment if it doesn't also result in a higher salary. Doing a three-year fellowship to save $60k is obviously a poor financial decision.

2. The bigger the difference between what you paid over 10 years and the amount you borrowed, the more PSLF saved you. People with long training will have the bulk of their loans forgiven.

3. Every year of training reduces the number of years you must make larger attending-sized payments by 1. You can easily calculate the worst-case scenario of each attending year by using the standard repayment for your loan amount, which is the most you would ever need to pay per month under PAYE or IBR. For $200,000, that was $2200 a month. For $300k, it's $3,331 a month. For $400k, it's $4,441. So, for each extra $100k you borrow, you could pay as much as $13,000 extra per year in the quest for PSLF.

The easiest way to do a quick comparison with some more personalized numbers is to use the free online calculator offered by Doctored Money at https://www.doctoredmoney.org/student-debt/loan-repayment-calculator. Fill it out like my chart above and you then can tweak marital status, children, etc. to see what repayment options will look like for different job possibilities, spousal employment, etc.

If you borrowed more than twice what you'll earn as an attending, PSLF is something you should really, really consider.

If you want to see how the hot dog is made, it's straightforward to do a quick back-of-the-napkin calculation to see if public service loan forgiveness is a viable choice for you. First, look at how many years you will be a resident or fellow. Take 9 and subtract it: that's the number of years you'll be making attending-sized payments. Why 9 and not 10? Because if all goes according to plan, there's a one-year lag between a salary increase and an IDR-payment-increase. Give yourself an average salary as a resident and give yourself an aver-age salary as an academic-type attending based on what you know about where you plan to do residency and where you may practice. Even though your salary will increase with each PGY-level and may increase each year as an attending, this is just to see if it's worth giv-ing more thought to. Add up ten years of payments and that's what it'll cost to get your loans forgiven.

In this case, we don't actually care what the "forgiven" amount is, because that number is higher as a result of low payments than it would've been if you'd been aggressive. All that is matters is how much money it takes to get out of debt. Any plan that requires actually paying off your debt will always cost more: the principal + the interest.

You may notice in so doing that the amount you pay is close to your actual loan amount. If so, going out of your way for PSLF is not for you; you'd easily make up the difference in the extra income from private practice. If your IDR payments don't cover accruing interest even as an attending, then PSLF will likely be a great deal for you regardless of the exact amount you will have forgiven.

Generally, people earning as much or more than owe each year with a short residency may not be impressed, whereas people in training for six or seven years will have more than half of their loans forgiven.

Every month of PSLF-eligible IDR you complete as a trainee is one less month of bigger payments you'll make as attending. Literally, anyone doing IDR in residency can have *some* of their loans forgiv-en. No amount of refinancing will get you to a negative interest rate of not paying the full amount you borrowed back!

COMPARING SALARIES BETWEEN JOBS

If you're an average borrower and can make IDR payments during training prior to working at a nonprofit after, PSLF will save you money *on your loans*. That's not debatable; it's just math. That doesn't mean PSLF makes academia magically more lucrative for most physicians than private practice in the long term. You'll have to weigh the money saved by PSLF versus the lost extra income from a more lucrative job. Remember, the purpose of the program was to incentivize people toward in-demand public service jobs that would otherwise be essentially unaffordable.

After years of school and training, you'll eventually land your first "real" job. If you've been doing your IDR throughout residency, you'll be well set up to either stay in academics and go for PSLF or consider the move to private practice.

Finding a job in the right place doing the right things with the right people is probably the most important goal.

But you'll still want to compare the benefits apples to apples, which means you'll want to take into account the PSLF-benefits in a non-profit vs the higher pay in practice.

The simplest way to do this is to calculate/guestimate how much total money you will need to pay to achieve PSLF for a nonprofit job vs how much you'll realistically need to pay off your loans in private practice (with or without private refinancing).

Take the difference between those two numbers and divide it by the number of years after graduating it'll take you to hit PSLF/10 years. That's essentially the tax-free PSLF salary bonus per year for that period of time.

So, compare your after-tax compensation from each job and add the PSLF bonus on to the academic one and see which comes out on top. Alternatively, subtract estimated taxes from the amount extra that private practice pays compared with nonprofit work and compare that to the PSLF bonus.

WHEN PSLF = BEING AGGRESSIVE

If paying your loans down quickly or going for PSLF are financially close to equivalent, then the safe choice is to actually pay off your loans. You never know what might happen to the government program or your life plans, but you do know that the faster you make payments and the more you put down, the more money you can save.

There are two reasons that paying down your loans may save you even more than one would think just running the numbers

- If you can refinance to a lower rate or can unexpectedly put more money toward your loans, then you can save even more.

- On the flip side, your PSLF quest can always get delayed by losing a month here or there and thus needing to pay extra, reducing PSLF's benefits. Or, you could even need to leave your full-time qualifying public sector work, throwing a big wrench in your plans.

RELYING ON THE GOVERNMENT

My feeling—and the feeling of most informed people without a vested interest in driving refinancing business—is that PSLF is a healthy plan for those who have already borrowed money but that its panacea status for combating ballooning medical school costs may not last forever. Our premedical colleagues starting a few years in the future may not be so lucky, and—given the bad press if nothing else—schools that rely on promoting this program to justify very large tuition raises will eventually need a reconciliation.

More discussion on the future of PSLF can be found in "The Future" chapter.

FINALLY

The best and most straightforward reason to plan to apply for PSLF is if you want to both train and practice at a non-profit or academic center. If so, doing your income-driven repayment (IDR) right is important.

As a resident, the best choice for most folks is to choose REPAYE and maximize that interest subsidy. REPAYE will allow most residents to have a low effective interest rate during training and give you the flexibility to either do PSLF efficiently or to double down as an attending and pay off your loans. That sounds a lot more fun than needing to pick a job you don't want just because your loans have tied your hands.

MAXIMIZING PSLF

If after the last chapter you're not interested in attempting to dedicate your limited financial energies to a program that may or may not exist forever, ignore this chapter. This is all about minimizing your payments made during the 120 months required to achieve loan forgiveness.

When it comes to PSLF, I advocate a trust-but-verify approach. As in, do everything possible to maximize PSLF, but don't use smaller monthly payments as an opportunity to blow extra dough on transient lifestyle goals. The best solution is to hedge your bets against a PSLF fallout by investing the difference: take any dollar you would have been spending toward your loans on the standard plan and put that toward retirement instead (or paying off other non-cancelable debts). This way, if PSLF were to suddenly disappear with no grandfathering or your employment circumstances change, you'd essentially have been investing on margin (i.e. investing with borrowed funds) and not just living your entire life with borrowed cash.

Because PSLF is a time-based program, if you can make smaller qualifying payments, then you will pay less money in total before your loan is forgiven. But also remember that outside of PSLF, making smaller payments means paying *more* for your loan over the long term because more interest accrues.

Minimizing payments to maximize loan forgiveness hinges on reducing the taxable income used to calculate your monthly payments. Because your IDR payment is based on 10-15% of your discretionary income, every dollar you can reduce your AGI by will reduce ("save") 10-15 cents the following year in payments.

Also note that in REPAYE, the same maneuvering to reduce your monthly payment will also consequently increase your interest subsidy, thus lowering your effective interest rate. All of this basically amounts to utilizing "above the line" deductions.

PRETAX RETIREMENT ACCOUNTS

Because contributing to pretax (not after-tax or "Roth") retirement accounts are the biggest and best way to reduce your taxable income, the PSLF program is essentially a subsidy on your retirement. You could consider it a partial non-employer "match."

Generally, most people would advocate using a Roth (after-tax) option as a resident if available because residents are likely to be a lower tax bracket than they will be in retirement. Roth contributions mean you pay taxes now but not when you use the money. Since you pay taxes on it now, these contributions do not reduce your taxable income and thus do not help you minimize loan payment amounts that will be wasted with PSLF. In this context, it's not necessarily straightforward to determine which option is best (tax bracket-related savings vs loan savings), but given current tax brackets, the traditional pretax option certainly isn't much worse than the benefits you'd expect from a Roth (unless tax brackets change substantially in the distant future).

For example, a resident earning $50,000 and contributing up to a 5% employer match would put $2,500 toward retirement and thus save $250 the following year in PAYE/REPAYE. A nice guaranteed return of 10% but perhaps not worth agonizing over. Starting good responsible financial habits and putting money away for retirement is the right move, no matter how you choose to do it. If you do have big side income (or your spouse is a high earner and you submit your taxes married filed jointly), then shielding this income from the IDR calculation will yield bigger savings.

Regardless, even if it's a wash for residents, it's almost certainly a good idea for high-earning attendings to go pretax, even if their employer-sponsored 401(k)/403(b) has a Roth option. In this context, your tax bracket is more likely the same or higher (making the Roth and pre-tax choices essentially equivalent), and you'll definitely get the 10-15% IDR partial match.

The annual contribution limit for a 401(k)/403(b) is $19,000 in 2019. Maxing that out would save you $1,800 the following year.

The annual contribution limit on a 457(b) account is also $19,000 in 2019. 457(b)s are common secondary pre-tax retirement accounts for government/state employees (and offered by an increasing number of regular nonprofits as well).

Maxing out both as an attending is a great thing to do to prepare for your future. Financial advisors call this *paying yourself first*, and it's an excellent idea whether you have loans or not. In the context of PSLF, it's even more excellent because maxing out these retirement accounts could save you $3800 in REPAYE/PAYE or $5,700 in IBR *each year* on top of keeping more of your money for yourself and less for Uncle Sam.

1099 INCOME (MOONLIGHTING, SOLOPRENEURSHIP)

If you make any money on the side as an independent contractor and not an employee (paid on a 1099 tax form instead of a W2), con-gratulations: you're a small business owner.

This is common for regular old moonlighting income but also for lo-cum tenens work, consulting, or even running a profitable website.

So, anyone earning any 1099 income is automatically running a business as the sole proprietor of a one wo(man) show. And that means you can also start a solo-401(k), an additional retirement ac-count for your small business of one. While the $19,000 personal limit is cumulative across all 401(k) accounts, your business can also contribute 20% of its profits to your 401(k) as well up to an annual maximum of $56,000 per account in 2019.

Essentially, if you made $10,000 moonlighting but had already maxed out your $19k contribution with your main work account, you could still basically put another $2,000 from that as an employer contribution. The details of setting that all up are beyond the scope of this book, but again—regardless of your loan situation—this is something to consider if the situation applies to you.

HSA ACCOUNTS

Health Savings Accounts are special investment accounts available to certain employees with high deductible health plans. The terms are so good that they're commonly referred to as "Stealth IRAs."

You put money into them like a 401(k) where it can be invested and grow tax-free. If you use the money for health expenses, you get to spend it tax-free as well. If you use it for anything else, you pay taxes on it like you would a traditional pretax retirement account.

Individuals can contribute $3,500 and married people can contribute $6,900 in 2019 for folks under the age of 55.

FLEX SPENDING ACCOUNTS

Putting money into a healthcare flexible spending account also reduces your pretax income, allowing you to pay for healthcare expenses tax-free (and also reducing loan payments). The downside to FSAs is that any money placed into one is a use-it-or-lose-it proposition, so don't put more money into one than you anticipate spending. These are particularly helpful when you have elective procedures or are having a child–things you can at least partially plan for in advance.

For people with dependents (children or adults), you can also put up to $4,000 in a dependent care flex account to pay for childcare/eldercare. Given how expensive daycare is, anyone with young children would have no problem maxing out this benefit. Some important limitations:

- Can't do it if you file taxes separately.

- Can't use it to pay a stay-at-home parent

- Can't use it to pay for actual school (like private K-12)

COLLEGE SAVINGS: THE 529

There are several tax-advantaged accounts to help parents saving for college. Of them, the 529 is the most popular and really the main one worth discussing.

The bottom line is that while 529s are great vehicles to save for college, contributions are *not* tax-deductible (for federal purposes) and thus will not save you any money for PSLF. Note that some states do provide a deduction for state taxes, however, which is nice even though it won't affect PSLF.

However, the growth in the account and the disbursements for educational expenses *are* tax-free, so parents should consider utilizing these once their traditional tax-advantaged retirement accounts have been maxed out (if they plan on helping their children pay for higher education).

In 2019, the 529 contribution limit is $15,000 per parent per child per year to avoid gift tax consequences. That's already a lot, but with multiple children, it adds up even faster. Even more egregious, parents can choose to "superfund" a 529 with five-years all at once for a maximum of $75,000 in a single year.

FINAL THOUGHTS ON INCOME-REDUCTION TECHNIQUES

After reading the above, you probably have mixed feelings:

On one hand, you can shield a goodly amount of money from your IDR calculation.

On the other hand, in order to do that you have to put the money in places where you can't blow it on fun things like new cars or vacations.

I hope after reading this far that you realize the latter is actually a good thing and will help keep you financially secure.

Between tax-advantaged accounts like the 403(b)/401(k), 457(b), HSA, and flexible spending accounts, a savvy borrower can reduce payments by thousands per year.

A dual income physician couple in academia with access to all of the above could put on the order of $80,000 away toward the future pre-tax and save over $8,000 each year in loan repayment for PSLF. If you were to do this immediately upon finishing training and have these funds withdrawn from your paycheck, you would never see this money nor feel this pain. It's very hard to grow into an income and spend money you don't have access to.

If you max out pre-tax accounts, consider setting up a loan payoff slush fund, where you'd place extra cash in an interest-bearing on-line savings account, CD, or even taxable investing account (for the risk-takers). While this jumbo emergency fund could be used for a home down payment or other large expense, it would also be available to help pay down loans quickly in case circumstances change. A backup plan is always a good thing to have.

MARRIED FILING SEPARATELY

You'll remember that in PAYE and IBR, married couples who file taxes separately are treated as individuals for purposes of calculating student loan payments.

You'll also remember that REPAYE closed this loophole and will account for both spouses' joint income regardless of filing status.

WHEN IS THIS HELPFUL FOR PSLF?

MFS is generally helpful when one spouse is high-income low-debt and the other (the one going for PSLF) is relatively low-income high-debt. The most common reason is basically residents with well-paid spouses, but any spousal pay will raise household income and thus payments.

That doc with the $200,000 loan and the $50,000 resident salary? What if their spouse had no debt and made $100,000 a year?

Filing jointly, the PAYE monthly payment would be $1,102.

Filing separately, the PAYE payment would be $268 (the same as a single resident).

You can see why people consider this a loophole. You could have a million-buck a year neurosurgeon spouse and still be paying pennies for loans as a resident and then get unlimited forgiveness years later.

CAVEAT: COMMUNITY PROPERTY STATES

Living in a community property state can complicate the MFS technique. The nine community property states are Arizona, California, Idaho, Louisiana, Nevada, New Mexico, Texas, Washington, and Wisconsin. In these states, married couples equally share in all income and assets they acquire after the wedding. This means that when filing taxes separately, you divide your total income by two instead of each filing for the fraction you actually contribute. For practical purposes, this has two scenarios:

1. If you make more than your spouse, then MFS in a community property state will lower your proportion of taxable income. This reduces your payments even more than normal (yay!).

2. If your spouse makes more than you, then MFS in a community property state will raise your proportion of taxable income. This reduces your payments less than normal (boo...).

Tax software or your friendly accountant can show you what your taxes will look like run both ways.

In scenario two, you might wonder if it is possible to then use pay stubs after MFS to more accurately reflect your real income? Yes (sometimes).

From the official IDR FAQ (#34):

> Q: *My spouse and I file separate federal income tax returns. However, we live in a community property state and are required to combine our incomes and split the total amount evenly for federal income tax reporting purposes. If I apply for an income-driven repayment plan, can my loan servicer consider only my individual income when determining my eligibility and payment amount?*
>
> A: *Your loan servicer may allow you to submit alternative documentation of your individual income that would be used instead of the AGI shown on your federal income tax return. Before you submit alternative documentation of your income, check with your loan servicer to see if this option is available.*

Remember that when using paystubs, your payments are calculated based on your income only and do not take into account deductions like retirement contributions. People occasionally fall into a trap of using pay stubs only to realize that their relatively decreased income is washed away by the inability to account for the deductions they were taking.

WHEN IS FILING SEPARATELY NOT HELPFUL?

When both spouses have similar income and debt levels or when the income differences are small overall. You'll often pay a few hundred to a few thousand more in taxes by filing separately, so the difference in loan payments should be more than a few bucks for you to try it.

HOW TO TELL?

The impact of joint/solo income on IDR is easy to calculate using the repayment estimator. The effect of MFS on taxes is harder to anticipate but can be done by running your taxes both ways in your tax software or with an accountant. Separate filings, for example, preclude taking the (wimpy) student loan interest deduction.

Moreover, MFS taxpayers must both claim the standard deduction, or must both itemize their deductions. Any extra itemized deductions for one spouse (examples below) may be offset the lack of itemized deductions for the other, though some of this will change with the new tax reform.

Tax breaks you lose when MFS (for the 2017 tax year):

- The child and dependent care tax credit (different from a dependent care flex account discussed above)

- The adoption credit

- The Earned Income Credit (not relevant for docs)

- Tax-free exclusion of U.S. bond interest

- Tax-free exclusion of Social Security benefits

- The credit for the elderly and disabled

- The deduction for college tuition expenses

- The student loan interest deduction

- The American Opportunity Credit and Lifetime Learning Credit for higher education expenses

- The deduction of net capital losses

- Traditional IRA deductions

On the plus side, outside of PAYE/IBR savings, there are several itemized deductions that are limited by adjusted gross income (AGI). These are easier to qualify when MFS because they will make up a larger percentage of a single spouse's income (particularly useful when the involved spouse is the one who makes less money):

- Medical expenses, deductible only to the extent they exceed 10% of AGI

- Personal casualty losses, deductible only to the extent they exceed 10% of AGI

- Miscellaneous itemized expenses, such as unreimbursed employee business expenses, fees for tax advice and preparation, and investment expenses, deductible only to the extent they exceed 2% of AGI

Note that for the latter, if you do any moonlighting or have any 1099 income, many of these income-limited deductions would be fully deductible as business expenses and thus not relevant. There are some serious perks to having even a relatively token amount of 1099 income.

If you save more in IDR payments over a 12-month span than it costs in taxes to file separately, then you should file separately from a PSLF-perspective. This may change year to year and should be re-evaluated every year come tax time.

IMPORTANT NUANCE: THE PAYE + REPAYE MFS COMBO FOR COUPLES

That's a mouthful, but there is a potentially huge nuance for couples where both partners have significantly different debt-to-income ratios (unbalanced income vs loans), such that the MFS loophole can work for or against you depending on which plan you choose.

Imagine you and your spouse are doing MFS to lower payments for a high-debt low-earning spouse in PAYE (or IBR) as usual, but the other (high-income low-debt spouse) opts for REPAYE instead.

For the spouse in PAYE, their loans and their income are treated separately as expected.

For the spouse in REPAYE, their payment is calculated as we discussed in the prior Income-Driven Repayment chapter: a total monthly payment based on household income *distributed proportionally based on the loan sizes.*

That's the key. Imagine you are the spouse with the high income and small loans. In PAYE MFS, you'd have a huge payment because of your high-income. But in REPAYE, the bulk of that payment would be *calculated* to go your spouse's loans (even though they're using the MFS loophole!). This can result in a much much lower monthly payment, since you only pay the fraction of that large household payment earmarked for your smaller loan.

If you and your spouse both have loans with different debt-to-income ratios, you need to run your numbers with the different plan combination possibilities in one of the calculators listed at the end of the book. What may be best for an individual may not always result in the lowest payments for the *household!* A spouse with a low debt-to-income ratio may leverage their spouse's high DTI to *lower* their payments by using REPAYE to ignore the very same MFS loophole that their spouse is using in PAYE. Absurd? You bet!

AVOID FRAUD

FedLoan has been known to occasionally tell borrowers in IBR or PAYE who have correctly filed their taxes separately that they need to check a box saying that they are "married but cannot reasonably access [their] spouse's information" on their annual income certification in order to utilize MFS. This is not true. That box was provided to help estranged spouses or sufferers of domestic violence. If you get this advice, ask for a supervisor.

SPOUSAL REFINANCE CAN AFFECT PSLF

As a reminder, if you refinance your loans you cannot get them forgiven.

It's also true that a spouse utilizing private refinancing can affect the PSLF-hopeful borrower. Two-loan couples will usually be MFJ, but if one refinances, suddenly their joint income is unchanged but their "debt" is drastically decreased because the **feds only consider federal loans in their IDR calculations**. That same-sized IDR payment would now be due just for the one loan, and you could even lose your partial financial hardship. If one spouse plans on refinancing, the other should be prepared to switch from REPAYE to PAYE and file separately.

Therefore, filing jointly and going for forgiveness together if you both have qualifying work may be a better option than filing separately and only one spouse refinancing or paying it down since there are tax costs to filing separately.

AMENDING PRIOR TAX RETURNS

If you want to be aggressive, you can have the best of both worlds. Changing your tax filing status from separate to joint (but not vice versa) is one of the reasons the IRS allows you amend prior tax returns. Amending a prior return is a paper process, so you'll usually need to download actual tax software (like Turbotax) in order to generate the amended returns or have an accountant do it for you.

You have three years from the original filing date to submit your amended return. Since all you're doing is changing filing status, it actually isn't all that complicated. In doing so, you can get the IDR benefits of MFS while recouping the initial tax losses after the fact by refiling MFJ. Sound shady? Totally, but there's literally nothing saying you can't.

TIMING YOUR INCOME RECERTIFICATION

We've covered this before, but it's important so we'll repeat it:

To remain in IDR, you must certify your income at least annually, but you don't have to do it at the exactly the same time. You can do it early when it suits you.

In short, you want to consider recertifying *whenever your income goes down*.

So, if you file together with your spouse who quits their job, is going part-time, on medical leave, etc., then recertify! The main caveat here is if you extensively utilize deductions to reduce your AGI; you may be required to use pay stubs to document your current income if it's before you have a new tax return demonstrating the change–which would be fine–except that it's possible to have your new lower salary be *higher* than your old higher salary minus deductions like retirement contributions. These machinations are things to do to save lots of money, not to shave off a few cents.

Conversely, if your income is about to increase, then the old advice was that you should also try to recertify early. For example, let's say you're normally due in August but are finishing residency in June and starting a new job in July. With the language of the old form, in order to be honest when you check that box saying your income hasn't changed, you would file in June before that new job starts. Again, how closely will the Department of Education audit borrowers? Who knows? But with potentially hundreds of thousands of dollars per borrower on the line, it wouldn't have surprised me if they figured out that doctors tend to start new jobs in July. Avoiding this issue entirely was one of the possible benefits of filing for a Direct Consolidation immediately after graduating. In 2019, they updated the form language to "income decrease," so now there is no reason to rush to rectify before a big pay raise.

Similarly, if you're about to get married to a working spouse, you may want to certify before you have a tax return reflecting the marriage. If you're about to get married to a non-working spouse, certify after and increase your family size. Again, note that your family size *should* include an unborn baby that is estimated to be born during the year.

LONG-TERM LOAN FORGIVENESS

If you've heard about getting your loans discharged after 20 years (PAYE) or 25 years (REPAYE/IBR), you should probably forget about it. Unless you quit medicine and never make a decent attending salary, all but those with the most egregious student loan amounts won't get their loans forgiven this way. Even if you did, you wouldn't save much money given all of those extra years of making payments.

Once you make good money, the calculated PAYE or IBR payment is capped at the equivalent of the standard 10-year repayment. If you make little enough (e.g. part-time academic primary care) to stretch out your loans for 20 years but couldn't do PSLF, then you might have some amount forgiven, but then you would have spent a ton of extra money over the years on interest, and the forgiven amount is taxed at your marginal tax rate. The best reason to keep your federal loans around at a high interest rate is generally for PSLF or because you can't yet qualify for something better.

THE TAX BOMB

As we've discussed previously, the 20/25-year loan forgiveness baked into income-driven repayment is taxable. While achieving PSLF would be a beautiful tax-free miracle, earning IDR forgiveness will result in a big potentially-unexpected tax bomb. The less you managed to pay over two decades and the more that's forgiven, the bigger that hit will be.

Let's say your debt entering repayment was $500,000 at 6% (an egregious amount as alluded to above). This accrues $30k per year in interest. Under PAYE, you need a salary of $310,000 in order to just break even on that interest. Thus, it's not that hard to imagine a scenario where that whole half mil gets forgiven after 20 years. And voila, you suddenly owe $140k in taxes (on top of paying over half a million bucks over the two decades to get there).

INSOLVENCY

Forgiven debt may be excluded from taxable income if the tax-payer is deemed insolvent, which is when their total liabilities exceed their assets.

Most physicians, even ones forced to stretch out their loans over two decades, will not be insolvent. Your house, retirement accounts, etc. all count as assets. But someone living in a rented abode and spending every dollar they earn or who is status post messy divorce could find themselves insolvent depending on how grotesque their student loan situation is. An accountant would be necessary here.

TAXES

The key facet of long-term loan forgiveness is that the forgiven amount is treated as income. This means that it may or may not be taxed at higher rates depending on your income that year (i.e. what bracket you are in). If you can reduce your income in the tax year that you earn forgiveness, such as maxing out pretax retirement accounts, you might be able to reduce the percentage taxed from the forgiven amount.

One way is simply to make less money in the year you'll be claiming loan forgiveness. Unlike PSLF, there are no employment requirements for IDR loan forgiveness, just the total number of on-time monthly payments. For example, if you have always wanted to spend a year working for Doctors without Borders or taking a sabbatical, this might be the year to do it. If you decide to leave the US and work abroad, around the first $100k of your income may fall off your tax return due to the Foreign Earned Income Exclusion.

(And if you just read that and realized that you could flee the country after graduating and use that exclusion to potentially never pay any money toward your loans until the tax bomb, that's true: call it the Expat Loophole.)

So, you'll still need to have enough money saved up to pay your taxes, but the marginal rate may be much less. In fact, it's not that you can't work, it's that you want to work only so far as the addition of your student loan "income" does not push you deep into a higher marginal tax bracket and result in a much greater fraction of the forgiven debt being taxed at a higher percentage.

FILING SEPARATELY

Filing your taxes separately in the forgiveness year also may be a smart move if you have a massive loan, as it may shield your spouse's income from a significantly higher bracket if you have a large forgiven amount.

Handling these sorts of issues is a rare case where a good accountant could make all the difference. At the very least, plugging it all into tax software and running it both ways would be mandatory.

THE MASSIVE DEBT CONUNDRUM

When PSLF won't work, the decision for massive debt is usually between refinancing and paying it down vs. paying the absolute minimum for 20-25 years and having it forgiven.

The decision-making here is more complex because you have to make some serious assumptions about your future, including what your income will be like for a very long time. Psychologically, you also need to figure between having some lean years initially in order to pay it off relatively quickly vs. make more payments over the course of at least two decades.

Again, when performing this calculus, you need to anticipate paying taxes on the forgiven amount. In this case, imagine the scenario in which you owe $400,000 at 6% in debt and essentially only make interest payments throughout your entire professional career while using income-driven repayment (e.g. salary of $260,000 in PAYE). In the case where you are magically exactly covering interest accrued and have $400,000 forgiven, you are now liable to pay the taxes due on this massive windfall come April the following year. 34% of $400,000 is a lot of money ($136k), so you'll even need to save money on the side (probably for years) just to deal with the tax consequences. You'll want to invest this money in order for it grow and have those dollars work harder for you. While this is doable, please know that it is not ideal. Then again, neither is being $400,000 in debt to begin with.

PAYE VS REPAYE

Before we get into the merits of PAYE vs REPAYE for 20/25-year forgiveness, let's remember: if you can get your loans forgiven via PSLF, then all of this is irrelevant and you'd save a ton of money. Your goal for PSLF should be to pay as little as possible per month during the 120 required monthly payments. It's not hard to imagine a 20-year plan that somehow squeezes 10 years of PSLF-qualifying payments into it.

But what about that person who borrowed $500,000 but wants to work part-time making $150,000 forever?

In this example, your salary is never big enough to pay more than the accrued interest, so you'd think REPAYE wins. A $500k loan at 6.8% accrues $34k in interest each year. The monthly payment at a $150k salary is $1102 ($13,224/year), meaning your loan continues to grow big time forever via negative amortization. You never lose your partial financial hardship—thus making the PAYE interest capitalization cap irrelevant—but the interest subsidy with REPAYE will significantly reduce the growth of the loan (and subsequently the tax you would owe when forgiven). Unfortunately, the wrinkle is in the extra five years you would need to qualify for forgiveness: 20 years in PAYE vs 25 years in REPAYE or IBR.

With a starting salary of 150k generously increasing at 5% per year, the federal repayment estimator projects PAYE forgiveness of $728k after 20 years and REPAYE $559k after 25 years while making payments of $451k for PAYE and $656k for REPAYE. At around a 35% average tax for that sum, for example, that's a tax bill of $255k for PAYE and $196k for REPAYE for the forgiven amount due in one big lump sum. Combine the total payments plus the forgiveness tax bomb and that's a total of $706k with PAYE and $852k with REPAYE. Because REPAYE takes longer, you pay $146k more with REPAYE. With either one, you'll need to save for years just to pay the taxes that will come due with the forgiveness (and even with your loans "forgiven," you're still spending a ton of money on them).

So that's the long-term scenario in which PAYE beats REPAYE for a single filer or non-working spouse: purely due to the 5 fewer years to qualify. But as always, these calculators make assumptions that might not be true nor reflect all of your options.

In this scenario, you'd theoretically maximize your benefits by being in REPAYE as long as you have an interest subsidy and then switching to PAYE while still eligible once you earn too much for the subsidy (if PAYE-eligible in the first place, of course). In this case, you'd get the best of both worlds: your months in REPAYE should still count toward the 240 payments needed for PAYE forgiveness, but you're also decreasing the amount of interest accrued as much as possible. If your REPAYE payments are never able to cover interest while in REPAYE, you'd stay in REPAYE until you near the 240 months needed for PAYE and then switch right before.

If you're married and your spouse works, then you need to use a calculator to see if your higher REPAYE payment (hopefully still with a subsidy) is better or worse than a lower PAYE payment without a subsidy coupled with any additional tax hits from filing separately. The bigger your loan and the less your spouse earns, the more likely the former is better.

If switching deviously like that sounds too good to be true, see #28 from the official FAQ:

> *Similarly, if you were previously in repayment under one income-driven repayment plan and later switched to a different income-driven repayment plan, payments*

you made under both plans will generally count toward the required years of qualifying monthly payments for the new plan.

Your servicer may not agree, but servicers are often completely wrong. See an analogous verbiage within the actual REPAYE regulations (page 67222 [yes, really]):

The statutory provisions that govern the ICR plans (which include the Pay As You Earn repayment plan, the ICR plan, and the REPAYE plan) and the IBR plan specify the types of payments that may be counted toward loan forgiveness under these plans. Generally, qualifying payments are limited to those made under one of the income-driven repayment plans, the standard repayment plan with a 10-year repayment period, or any other plan, if the payment amount is not less than the payment that would be required under the standard repayment plan with a 10-year repayment period.

It's probably worth discussing this with your servicer before you a make a decision that might haunt you two decades in the future. No one has done this yet because no one is even close to hitting the 20-year mark, let alone in clever ways.

And lastly, it's again worth noting that while 20 years is a leisurely payment schedule, you'd probably still spend less money just paying it down faster. Refinancing that same $500k loan even to 5% with a 10-year term would cost you around $636k to pay off (though it would admittedly also cost you $5000 a month, ouch). Don't forget that all it takes is a bump in your salary to totally throw off your clever plan. Get that new rate down to 4% and you're looking at closer to $607k. The bottom line is that most physicians won't be saving actual money by going for long-term forgiveness; they're merely spreading out the suffering.

You might feel that you'd rather take the extra money it would take to pay off your loan and invest it yourself instead. Investing on margin is a risky proposition, and you'll never be guaranteed a return better than the current student loan interest rates. It's probably reasonable to do this in the context of tax-advantaged retirement accounts, which have annual contribution limits. It's a bit riskier to do this in a taxable account without any extra benefits to account for the risk. Maxing out accounts like a 401(k), 403(b), 457(b), or (likely "Backdoor") Roth IRA is one thing, especially as pretax contributions also reduce AGI and IDR payments. Doubling down on a taxable account doesn't have these multi-pronged benefits.

As always, you'll have to run some scenarios for yourself, but if you're considering long-term long forgiveness, hopefully this gives you some food for thought.

OTHER FORGIVENESS & LOAN REPAYMENT PROGRAMS (LRP)

Note that many programs offering repayment assistance (like the VA) are also government work and thus qualify for PSLF.

JOB-RELATED REPAYMENT/STIPENDS

Some employers offer student loan repayment as a bonus package for new employees. In many cases, these payments are made directly to the servicer on your behalf and are considered a taxable benefit. This is great, and you should enjoy that perk *unless* said employer is also a non-profit 501(c)(3) organization and you are otherwise well-suited for PSLF. In this case, you'll be paying taxes on money that would have been forgiven anyway. For example, a $20,000 loan repayment benefit costs $5,600 in taxes in the 28% bracket!

In the context of PSLF, a taxable student loan benefit is actually worse than nothing.

If this situation crops up during the negotiation/contact-signing phase, it behooves you to try to negotiate a change. If possible, try to get this money delivered to you instead of your servicer (then you can use it to make your IDR payments). Having them make it a retirement contribution would also be great if they don't want to just give you cash. Some big organizations are inflexible and won't/can't do anything helpful for you. If you're really set on PSLF and they won't play ball, you should try to waive the benefit. But otherwise, make sure that the extra money doesn't change the calculus. It's possible that with the bonus you'll be better off just trying to pay down the loans fast yourself instead of stretching over the 10-year span.

LOCAL & STATE PROGRAMS

Some states have their own loan repayment programs, typically reserved for those practicing in rural areas or taking care of underserved populations. Some of these are tied to seeing a certain number or percentage of Medicaid patients.

These programs aren't generally robust enough to change your plans, but if you're considering practicing in a more altruistic environment, make sure you look into your state's offerings.

VETERAN'S AFFAIRS

The VA offers up to a maximum of $10,000 per employee per calendar year up to a total of $60,000. Note that VA work is PSLF eligible.

NIH & NHSC

The National Institutes of Health (NIH) has programs that supply up to $35k per year. See https://www.lrp.nih.gov/eligibility-programs:

> *The repayment amount is equal to one-quarter of the total eligible educational debt, up to $35,000, for each year of the award. To receive the maximum amount of $70,000 for a two-year award, an applicant must have at least $140,000 in eligible educational debt at the contract start date.*

The National Health Service Corps (NHSC) offers loan repayment up to $50k in exchange for a two-year commitment. See http://nhsc.hrsa.gov/loanrepayment/.

Both of these require competitive applications and acceptance is certainly not guaranteed.

STUDENTS TO SERVICE PROGRAM

For medical students in their last year of school, the NHSC offers a Students to Service Program that provides up to $120,000 toward educational costs and student loans.

In return, the med student commits to provide primary health care at an NHSC-approved site for three years after graduation.

THE MILITARY

Military benefits are great if you were planning on serving your country anyway and your primary goal is to take care of soldiers and their families.

Prospectively, you can choose one of the military's HSPS programs (Health Professionals Scholarship Program) to pay for medical education in exchange for service as a commissioned officer. You enter the military match and all that entails and pay back each year of service after residency.

Contrast that with the various military Financial Assistance Programs (FAP), which help you pay for medical school after the fact. You pick and finish your school, land your civilian residency and then get the financial support as a trainee. You owe one year of service for each year you receive assistance, plus an additional year.

The numbers aren't as pretty when you consider reduced pay as an attending compared to civilian life and lack of autonomy, especially for those with families. FAP allows you to delay the decision to enter the military if you're unsure, as a lot of HSPS enrollees without prior service experience regret their decisions. But years of obligated service add up fast regardless of which program you enter.

As a medical school payment vehicle, the military is certainly not perfect. The more you borrow and the lower paid your specialty, the better deal HSPS will be. Expensive private school and primary care? Pretty good deal. State school orthopedist? Not so much.

ARMY

The Army's Financial Assistance Program offers grants up to $45k per year along with a monthly stipend of at least $2,000 to army members during residency.

The Active Duty Health Professions Loan Repayment Program offers up to $120k ($40k over 3 years) towards repaying medical school loans for active duty doctors.

Health Professionals Special Pay offers up to $75k ($25k over 3 years) to both active duty physicians and doctors who are members of the U.S. Army Reserve who have completed a residency in a qualifying specialty.

NAVY

The Navy's Health Professions Loan Repayment Program (HPLRP) offers a yearly maximum payment of $40,000 directly to medical school loans, after federal income taxes that are typically about 25 percent. This is open to active duty medical students, residents, and attending physicians.

The Navy Financial Assistance Program offers up to $275k in assistance to medical residents ($45k/year) as well as a monthly stipend of at least $2,200 for four years.

The Navy also advertises sign-on bonuses to practicing physicians of $220k -$400k, depending on the physician's specialty and experience.

AIR FORCE

The Air Force will pay for medical school through its Health Professions Scholarship Program.

For those joining later, the Air Force Financial Assistance Program offers grants up to $45k per year with a monthly stipend of $2,000.

INDIAN HEALTH SERVICES LOAN REPAYMENT PROGRAM

Working in an IHS facility for American Indians and Alaska Natives for two-year commitments can net $40k in medical school loan repayment.

FEDERAL LOAN DISCHARGE

There are handful of depressing ways to have your loans discharged (cancelled)

- All of your loans are cancelled in the event of death or total permanent disability (i.e. you cannot and will never be able to work)

- Bankruptcy is theoretically possible, but not really. If you can work, the bankruptcy court is not going to let you off the hook.

- Closed School (basically only for folks who could not complete their program because the school closed while they were enrolled)

- Loans were the result of identity theft

- False Loan Certification (the school lied to make you eligible for loans)

PRIVATE REFINANCING

While medical school is expensive and getting more so every year, federal student loans are still earning the government a tidy sum (at least those actually being repaid). Combine the two and a new doctor will borrow more and then pay more for the privilege than at any other time in history.

Over the past few years, historically low-interest rates and a rebounding economy have led private banks to re-enter the student loan business, particularly on the refinancing side. Student loan refinancing/consolidation is exactly what it sounds like: the refinancing company or bank pays off all of your current loans and creates a single loan in its place that they hold at a new interest rate. Their profits come from all the interest you'll be paying to them instead of the feds or other banks. Because banks borrow money at super low rates (recently as low as 0%), they can still make money refinancing borrowers at comparatively low rates. Refinancing is not altruism, even though it's recently worked out well for student loan borrowers. It's just a rare market opportunity that can actually benefit consumers.

INTEREST RATE IMPACT ON A $200,000 LOAN WITH 10-YEAR REPAYMENT

INTEREST RATE	MONTHLY PAYMENT	TOTAL INTEREST PAID
6.8%	$2,302	$76,193
6.5%	$2,271	$72,515
6.0%	$2,220	$66,449
5.5%	$2,171	$60,463
5.0%	$2,121	$52,447
4.5%	$2,073	$48,732
4.0%	$2,025	$42,988
3.5%	$1,978	$37,326
3.0%	$1,931	$31,746
2.5%	$1,885	$26,248

In 2015, when the student loan refinancing game heated up and companies first started offering plans specifically tailored towards residents, refinancing should have been a no-brainer for a significant fraction of residents and every attending not considering PSLF. Unfortunately, at the time, very few people knew these options even existed. As you can see in the table, a lower rate makes a big difference.

Now, the landscape has shifted again. First, newer borrowers have lower federal interest rates than the usual 6.8%+ older borrowers had. Then the government's new REPAYE program reduced the effective interest rate for many residents. While refinancing is still an excellent option for many attendings, it is no longer the best plan even for most non-PSLF-bound residents, at least those who qualify for a nice REPAYE subsidy and are willing to make income-based payments. For those non-PSLF-bound who are currently forbearing or planning to forbear, looking into refinancing with a resident-friendly company is still definitely worth considering; in most cases, you'll save money.

Overall, I remain surprised at how little most of these companies have done to court doctors. I don't care how well Peter is doing as a junior associate at BankCorp, I refuse to believe he's as much of a sure bet as even a resident physician, full stop. Doctors at every stage of training are reliable people with large loans and a near guarantee of paying them off.

GENERAL CONSIDERATIONS WHEN REFINANCING

Interest rates are always advertised as a range. The shorter the term, the lower your debt-to-income ratio, and the better your credit score, the better the rates you'll actually receive when you apply to private companies. These companies are looking for borrowers with good credit histories, proof of a stable income, and enough cash flow to support their monthly loan payments.

If you don't qualify or don't get a good rate by yourself, you can consider applying with a cosigner. This means that the second party is now also responsible for your loans if you drop the ball for any reason. Additionally, the cosigned loan will show up on their credit report and can affect their ability to get loans or mortgages of their own. Some companies do offer co-signer release opportunities after a set period of on-time payments, as fast as after one year, but this may or may not be something you're willing to consider.

Choosing a variable instead of a fixed rate will also get you a better rate, but that's your upfront reward for taking on the risk of rates going up in the future. Some people do get the lowest possible advertised rate (often derisively called the "teaser rate"), but most do not.

Examples of the effect of term rate and term length on total repayment:

	5 YEAR	10 YEAR	15 YEAR	20 YEAR	25 YEAR
LOAN BALANCE	$200,000	$200,000	$200,000	$200,000	$200,000
INTEREST RATE	3%	4%	5%	5.50%	6%
MONTHLY PAYMENT	$3,594	$2,025	$1,582	$1,376	$1,289
TOTAL INTEREST	$15,624	$42,988	$84,686	$130,186	$186,581
TOTAL PAYMENT	$215,624	$242,988	$284,686	$330,186	$386,581

Divide the amounts in the chart by whatever number it takes to get to your actual loan amount for a more personal illustration (so if you borrowed $50k, divide the monthly repayment and total interest by 4).

Effect of the just term length on total repayment:

	5 YEAR	10 YEAR	15 YEAR	20 YEAR	25 YEAR
LOAN BALANCE	$200,000	$200,000	$200,000	$200,000	$200,000
INTEREST RATE	5%	5%	5%	5%	5%
MONTHLY PAYMENT	$3,774	$2,121	$1,582	$1,320	$1,169

TOTAL INTEREST	$26,455	$54,557	$84,686	$116,779	$150,754
TOTAL PAYMENT	$226,455	$254,557	$284,686	$316,779	$350,754

When comparing interest rates to your current federal loans, you should also consider capitalization, which can be substantial after a few years of negative amortization. Your current federal loan accrues interest on the current principal, but the new refinanced loan's principal will be the combination of the current principal *and* all of the accrued interest.

A $200,000 loan at 6% accrues the same interest per year as a $240,000 loan at 5%: $12,000. That $40,000 difference could easily accrue during training, and thus refinancing to 5% in this scenario wouldn't actually save you money.

Since cash flow is important, trading a federal loan (with its possibility of forbearance or IDR) for a private loan may not be a good idea right before buying a house, depending on the size of your mortgage and student loans, as the underwriters may not be as confident that you can make mortgage payments on top of a large fixed student loan payment. This is most commonly an issue for people trying to buy a house during residency, especially at the beginning. Of course, if you're buying a reasonably priced house for your income, this should be less of an issue. This also wouldn't be an issue if your monthly payment size isn't changing significantly.

VARIABLE VS FIXED

While variable rates are always cheaper at the beginning than fixed rates, they don't always stay that way. They can get even better (sometimes), but in a world of recent historically low interest rates, they can also go up. These rates are usually tied to some external measure of bank borrowing such as the LIBOR, and each company will have their own maximum rate and sometimes a maximum rate of change. These are always available to you before you sign anything but are important when considering your options.

In general, if you're an attending who could afford to pay off your loans in a few years and who has the financial flexibility to increase the money flowing toward your loans if needed, in many cases, you'll be better off with the variable rate. You'll enjoy the savings off the bat, and if rates go up, then you push harder and pay them off as fast as possible. If you can afford a 5-year variable term, then go for it. Even if rates go up, it takes some time to undo the savings.

If you're looking at years and years of payments no matter what you do, then the risk probably isn't worth it.

Ideally, a new attending would pick a 5-year (or shorter) term variable loan and be prepared to knock it down faster if needed. Otherwise, a 10-year fixed loan is a reasonable option. No company has prepayment penalties, so you can always pay it down faster. And, because these are also no-cost refinances, there's nothing to stop you from rate shopping when rates go down and refinancing again, even with the same company.

LOST PROTECTIONS & BENEFITS

All those websites and advisors promoting refinance will allude to vague protections of federal loans that you'll lose if you refinance privately. These are what matters:

1. Obviously no PSLF. Refinancing is for people who actually need to pay down their debt.

2. No income-driven repayment. Except for companies which offer a reduced monthly payment during residency, payments are based on a length of time, not your income. This matters if you anticipate big swings in your income such that you might not be able to make big payments consistently. This is less of an issue for most docs.

3. No forbearance. Sort of. Many companies offer brief periods of forbearance on the order of a few months.

4. Did I mention **no loan forgiveness**? You can refinance over and over again, but you can never ever go back to the feds once you leave.

MYTHS

Private lenders come after your family if you die.

Private lenders demand their money back even if you're permanently disabled.

Frankly, those would be deal breakers for most people. And, contrary to a lot of people's assumptions, they generally aren't true.

These are both important protections of federal loans. In the competitive market for student loan refinance, the *majority* of companies have followed suit and guaranteed the same protections. **Definitely read the fine print before you sign anything**; most but not all companies publicize terms and stipulations that mirror the feds. But in particular, if you need to use a cosigner, find out if they'll be on the hook if you die or become disabled—this would be the sneaky pitfall.

INTEREST CAPITALIZATION

Capitalization is a big pitfall for borrowers when considering refinancing.

One thing that happens with any private refi is that your accrued interest will capitalize. This means that if you had loans of $180k with $40k of accrued interest, your new loan amount (that will now be gaining interest) is $220k after refinancing. That sounds bad, but it all depends on the numbers:

$180k at 6.8% accrues $12,240 every year in interest. $220k at 5.6% accrues $12,320 the first year in interest.

What this illustrates is that you can't just compare the two rates apples to apples if you have unpaid interest. You need to compare the combination of the interest rate with the loan amount and see how much interest accrues every year.

Also note that interest capitalizes anyway at end of your six-month grace period after finishing school, when you file for a Direct Consolidation loan, or after a period of forbearance, so this is irrelevant if one of these events has happened recently.

What *would* always be relevant is any private loan's capitalization interval, if any. All loans' interest rates are marketed as APR (annual percentage rate), which is basically just the interest rate (plus any fees wrapped in).

Every legitimate student loan company I know of uses simple interest without any capitalization during repayment, so the APR is an accurate reflection. Some other private loans may capitalize at some interval (as often as daily) and their rates would be more accurate if expressed as an APY (annual percent yield). In practice, this results in a small rate bump. You can use this calculator to convert the APR you receive to an APY that reflects compounding: https://mindyourdecisions.com/blog/apr-to-apy-converter/. (Note: in resident-specific refinance programs, your loans do capitalize at the end of your training period when you *begin* repayment but not again *during* repayment.)

For example, that 5.6% APR loan has an APY of 5.76% if compounding daily. The actual interest it will accrue would thus be $12,672.

Ultimately, the APY nuance isn't likely to be important in this particular rodeo, but it illustrates that you should get in the habit of reading the fine print whenever you sign anything, especially if it involves piles of money.

REFINANCING > FORBEARANCE

So, there are many benefits of federal student loans (income-driven repayment, the REPAYE interest subsidy, the possibility of PSLF), but none of them meaningfully apply if you don't enter into an income-driven repayment plan during residency. Forbeared loans are just loans that accrue a lot of interest at high rates. If you can switch to a private company and save a point or two on your rate during residency, you'd likely save thousands in interest during training.

The main exceptions are individuals with massive debt and plans for semi-permanent "relatively low" income. A person with $400,000 in loans with plans to enter academic pediatrics making $150k a year will still benefit from IDR programs and PSLF after forbearance, as he or she will essentially function as a resident forever from a debt-to-income perspective. Even the companies that have resident-friendly plans ask for your specialty, which they basically use as a proxy for future income before refinancing.

THE FEAR SCENARIO

The whole point of refinancing is to get a better rate than what you already have. The REPAYE interest subsidy makes this a bit more complicated because the most likely scenario is that a resident-friendly private company will offer you a rate that is better than your actual federal rate but worse than your current *effective* rate.

But, on the flip side, it's also possible that by the time you make enough money to lose a good effective REPAYE rate and want to refinance that the golden window has closed and private rates have gone up (that's what the lenders want you to think at least). I would argue that such prognostication is generally unsatisfying and as foolish as trying to time the market, especially for those just beginning training.

REFINANCING PRIVATE LOANS

If you already hold private loans, there's an excellent chance that their rates are higher than what companies are currently offering. Even if you're able to do IDR during residency, you should always look into refinancing any private loans. Again, refinancing is a no-cost proposition.

Once you hold any private loans, you should be checking the rates periodically to see if they've improved. If they have, refinance again.

REFINANCING AS A RESIDENT

If you're a resident with a boatload of student loans from the feds, your choice has historically been IDR or forbearance. The mountain of debt compared with your relatively paltry resident salary has put conventional student loan refinancing out of reach.

However, there are currently several companies that offer specific plans to residents which involve a reduced (e.g. $100/month) monthly payments during residency. The details are of course subject to change. See benwhite.com/refinancing for details.

While residents in their final year of training with a signed job contract can usually secure an "attending" rate, residents earlier in training won't be so lucky. In general, residents earning a REPAYE subsidy or without PLUS loans will not be particularly impressed. Again, most residents would do better to stick with IDR for their federal loans (although these programs would of course still be a good idea for those with private loans). Check out the URL above for the various program options and how they work.

Ultimately, the reduced monthly payments will make a private refi "cheaper" on a monthly basis than an IDR plan after the first year or two of training. The downside, of course, is that if you only make the minimum required monthly payments then you just accrue more interest. And interest capitalizes at the end of the training period when entering repayment (just like after a federal forbearance period). There are no prepayment penalties though, so if you can make bigger more-IDR-sized payments, then by all means do it. You can refinance as a resident and continue to make as big a payment as you can afford. And, of course, the more you pay now the more you save in the long run.

Most residents won't qualify for refinancing outside of a special resident program, because most trainees' debt to income ratio is far away from the underwriting requirements most companies use (i.e. they want you to make more per year than you owe, not owe four times what you make per year). It's a bummer that the rates offered to residents are not as good as those offered to attendings, so if you do apply as a resident but aren't impressed (or don't bother applying), that doesn't mean you should give up on the idea once you're out of training if you're not PSLF-bound. Attendings who aren't going for PSLF should basically all refinance and save thousands.

Lucky borrowers who have escaped with five-figure or low six-figure debt may be able to squeeze into a traditional private refinance which may land them better rates. As a general rule, if you can afford the standard 10-year repayment (i.e. you don't or barely have a partial financial hardship), then you might as well refinance once the private rate is better than your effective REPAYE rate. Since there are no costs or penalties, you can and should refinance again as an attending.

Ultimately, most residents should refinance any private loans but probably leave their Direct loans where they are.

WHAT ABOUT PSLF?

Keep in mind, PSLF can only take place after 10 years of monthly payments. The smaller your loan burden and the shorter your residency, the less you can theoretically have forgiven. PSLF is the best deal for those with long residencies/fellowships (low monthly payments for longer under IDR) and with a lot of loans (private school = more forgiven).

As an average attending, the desire to do PSLF is the main real reason to continue holding federal loans if you otherwise qualify for private refinancing. As a resident, REPAYE is likely better than refinancing and it keeps your options open. If you can afford the IDR payments, you should probably stick with the program.

REFINANCING JUST PLUS LOANS

If you have PLUS loans and are confident about PSLF not being for you, you may think it would be helpful to compare your effective RE-PAYE rate of both your regular Direct Unsubsidized loans as well as your PLUS loans to what you can get from a private company. You may then think that it's only worth refinancing your PLUS ones, but it's probably not. Your REPAYE payment is based on your current *income* and not on your debt amount. Thus, your IDR payments won't go down. That same amount will go to just your remaining federal loans, reducing the amount of unpaid interest and thus raising your effective interest rate. On top of that, you'll now have to make payments on that new private loan as well.

It may be worth refinancing a fraction of your loans if the effective interest rates are still above what private refinancing can offer, but it's unlikely to work well if you're benefiting from an interest subsidy.

FINAL THOUGHTS: REPAYE VS PRIVATE REFINANCING

If you consolidate at the end of school, you should hopefully be able to net zero-dollar payments for REPAYE and enjoy the fullest possible subsidy: the forgiven interest reduces your effective interest rate by half! No matter how much you borrowed and how much you'll make, anyone with $0 payments will get that subsidy. As a result, it's going to be hard to get a better rate your intern year. Once your payments really kick in, you may calculate that private refinancing is better. This is particularly common for those who managed to escape with five-figure or low six-figure debt. For the rest, REPAYE will likely still ultimately be the stronger choice during training, followed by private refinance once an attending (again, if not considering PSLF or for the unfortunate souls considering the 20/25-year IDR loan forgiveness). This assumes that you can afford and will pay that 10% monthly payment. Refinancing is generally better than forbearing for any significant amount of time (the exception is someone with very large loans but permanently low income, as we discussed in the chapter on Long-term Loan Forgiveness.

SHOULD A RESIDENT REFINANCE?

- If you have private loans at high rates, this is a no-brainer.

- If you have federal loans and have been forbearing, then this is also probably worth checking out. $100 a month to slow down the relentless climb of accruing interest could save thousands (but only if the rate is substantially lower, which it probably won't be)

- If you're doing IDR temporarily but planning to start forbearing (barely making ends meet now and having kids soon, etc.), then it only makes sense to refinance if you can afford the token payment.

- If you have federal loans and are doing IDR to be financially responsible but have no interest/faith in PSLF, then refinancing is also worth considering only if you're not getting much of a REPAYE subsidy. The "resident" rate is unlikely to beat your effective REPAYE rate but may beat the actual rate, particularly if you have PLUS loans. If you're married and are paying the fed's sticker rate, then a private company will probably save you some money there as well. As there is no prepayment penalty, you are free to still make your old IDR-sized payments (only now those payments will go a lot further at a lower interest rate). If you know you want to do private practice, then there's really no big reason to stick with IDR just for IDR's sake if it's costing you more.

- If you're in REPAYE but not considering PSLF, then feel free to apply for private refinance, but only pull the trigger if the rate you're offered is lowered than your effective interest rate with the REPAYE unpaid interest subsidy. This is unlikely.

- Keep in mind you'll get a better rate as a trainee if you are in your final year and have a signed employment contract.

- Residents with substantial loans probably shouldn't refinance regardless of your future plans, because those are just plans.

You don't know what kind of job you'll find after residency, and it would be really sad to miss out on PSLF just because you were cynical or overconfident.

APPLYING TO COMPANIES

The initial applications are short (really short, usually 5 minutes or less). Rate ranges are typically pretty similar across lenders (and all will typically advertise a rate with a 0.25% auto-debit discount factored in already) but idiosyncratic enough that you can't predict consistently which company will actually give you the best deal. The brief initial application will give you a preliminary rate and will not affect your credit score. The hard-pull on your credit comes when you actually move forward with official paperwork stuff. The credit bureaus also treat multiple pulls for the same reason to be comparison shopping, so you won't be penalized for applying to multiple companies at the same time—it'll just be the single hit on your credit.

The prudent thing for an attending or lucky resident to do is to apply for refinancing from each company that can theoretically meet your needs and see which one is willing to refinance you at the best rate.

When it comes time to apply for refinancing, you should assume pretty much any link you click online will be a referral link from which someone will make some money. The big websites like Student Loan Hero promote refinancing heavily because their income model is primarily based on refinancing referrals, which are worth hundreds of dollars apiece (and I'd venture pay-to-play featured placement for an additional fee). Smaller sites run by individuals (like mine) sometimes split those referrals with you. My referral links are available at benwhite.com/refinancing. That said, I'm not trying to be a shill for private refinance and referral commissions, so if this discussion makes you uncomfortable, by all means use someone else's links. Some of the lenders even offer open programs where you and your friends can refer each other. But since you can often get a few hundred bucks back through a referral, you might as well use someone's.

To keep this section short and timeless, I've left the ever-shifting details for each company online at benwhite.com/refinancing. If refinancing doesn't make sense for you, then you don't have to read it!

Overall, the interest rate ranges offered by these companies are generally comparable. Typically, when one lowers their rates, the others have followed quickly followed suit. The increasing competition in this space has generally been excellent for consumers, though the rate nadir seems to have already come and gone. Before REPAYE, private refinancing would have been a great choice for many residents and most attendings. Now, private refinancing is a great choice for a much smaller number of residents (but still a lot of attendings).

Again, if you have several potential options based on your loan burden and your income, you might as well apply to all and see who gives you the best deal. You can't predict ahead of time. Applications are relatively short and painless, so there isn't a big-time investment in doing your due diligence. If you've refinanced, make sure to check rates periodically (especially if the marketed ranges change, your credit score or income improves, etc.). Once you've pulled the trigger, don't shy away from refinancing over and over again if you can get a better rate. It never costs you anything, and you can keep racking up referral bonuses.

As an attending, unless you are making qualifying payments toward achieving some sort of loan forgiveness, there is little reason to stay with federal loans if you qualify for a better rate elsewhere. Being an attending making good money and actually paying off your loans means that you're unlikely to benefit from any of those great provisions of income-driven repayment. If you're not benefiting from those, then all you have is a loan with a high interest rate.

PAYING DOWN FASTER

Let's say you're one of the 60% of docs who plan to actually pay off your loans yourself. There are no "5 crazy tricks to blasting your student loans," but there are a few considerations to speed things up.

PAY MORE

Just pay more per month. It's that simple. Earmark more of your income toward paying down your debt and have it auto-debited from your account so you don't have a choice. If you're being clever, you could even have the necessary fraction of each paycheck routed via direct deposit to a different checking account and use that one for student loans—then you'll never even *see* the money. The key here, as advocated by Dr. James Dahle in *The White Coat Investor,* is to "live like a resident." That new attending income is there so you can pay yourself first. That means student loans and retirement before fancier cars and bigger houses.

WHERE TO PUT IT

Federal loan servicers are required to use any extra payments to pay down any accrued interest first. Then, they're supposed to put any principal payments toward the highest-interest debt. However, they occasionally don't and spread it evenly. If there's any leeway for a human being to make a bad decision on your account, just take the extra time to be clear. You can always specify where you want extra payments to go, and you want them to go toward your highest-interest debt. If you have a consolidation loan or all of your loans have the same rate, then you're set already. (Did I mention you really don't want to have credit card debt? Take care of that first.)

Once you've paid accrued interest, it's time to be extra clear:

1. Make a separate payment from your monthly payment

2. Tell them which loan(s) you want it to go to

3. Tell them not to "advance your due date" or whatever other way they specify to make this an extra voluntary payment to be applied now and not earmarked for future required payments

4. Follow up to make sure they did what you asked

Whenever making an extra payment, you'll have the choice to "advance your due date" or keep your next automatic payment as scheduled. Advancing the due date means your payment will be used to cover next month's payment. If your goal is to pay your loan faster, you do not want to advance the due date—you want extra payments, not just early ones.

LEVERAGING OTHER DEBT

In the Borrowing Less chapter, we already discussed leveraging debt a bit, but the basic idea is simple: use debt at a lower interest rate to pay off debt with a higher interest rate and thus save money in the process. Whenever you consider any "debt reshuffling," make sure to consider any associated fees. It's easy for loan origination or transaction fees to wipe away benefits.

Also note that no matter the difference in interest rates that there is a potentially important unanticipated risk: student loans are discharged on death or permanent disability. Personal loans, credit cards, mortgages, etc. are not. On the other hand, you can discharge pretty much every other kind of debt during bankruptcy... except for student loans.

THE MORTGAGE

In addition to hopefully having a lower rate, interest paid on a mortgage is generally 100% tax-deductible (if you itemize), which can make a big difference (student loan interest is basically not, especially for attendings; we'll discuss that in the next chapter on Taxes). There are two main ways to use a home as a vehicle to help pay off your student loans:

REFINANCE A HOME YOU ALREADY OWN OR TAKE A HOME EQUITY LOAN

A cash-out refinance will almost always have a better rate, though you generally have low to no closing costs on a home equity loan (sometimes called a second mortgage). If rates are lower now than when you got your mortgage, refinancing is going to be an even better idea. If you're moving soon, a home equity line may be better due to lower up-front costs.

Price out both options. Both are easier to do if your house is worth substantially more than you owe on it, and both may be more complicated depending on underwriting requirements. It's not uncommon to need to use a "physician loan" product to get a mortgage as a young doc with a lot of loans.

GET A BIGGER LOAN THAN YOU NEED ON A NEW HOME

If you buy a fixer-upper, for example, you might take out a bigger loan ostensibly for the purposes of renovation and use the extra to pay off your loans.

WORTH IT?

Any mortgage fun will depend on the price of the loan versus the appraised value of your home. And before jumping the gun, remember that closing costs on a mortgage (new or refinanced) are non-zero. A new loan may also often have an origination fee on top of any closing costs.

Some lenders love this idea—SoFi even advertises a student loan payoff/mortgage financing combo package (though unsurprisingly the student loan portion of the package isn't the most generous).

CREDIT CARDS

You can't use a credit card to directly pay your servicer, but you can use an intermediary service like Plastiq, which we discussed in detail in the Borrow Less Chapter. You can occasionally even use those balance transfer checks that your card company won't stop sending you in the mail. Neither of these comes free, and in most cases, you don't even earn points/miles/bonuses on balance transfers (please, read the fine print, those checks are generally a terrible idea). Depending on the amounts at play and the rate of interest accumulating on your loans, it's quite possible that the fees involved will be a wash with the interest savings—but then you'll get the points to make it "worthwhile." Also note that you'll only save money on interest accumulation if the extra cash is enough to go to the principal. Paying a fee to pay off interest itself isn't going to do you any good.

Any scheme leveraging credit cards basically amounts to point-hacking. There are blogs and blogs dedicated to this practice: which cards to use, how to manufacture spending to get rewards, which loopholes are still open for which companies. It can be time-consuming. It definitely isn't for everyone. It isn't even for most people. If these ideas excite you, it's crucial you do your due diligence: miscalculating a perk can easily end up costing more than you were ever going to save. Never carry a balance past the introductory term.

PERSONAL LOANS

Personal loans are almost always at a higher rate than both your student loans or any secured debt (e.g. mortgage) you have. You probably don't want personal loans.

Ditto "Practice Loans," which while often better than your average personal loan, still aren't going to be that great.

TERMS

Reshuffling your debt to a lower interest rate but a longer term isn't going to save you much money; it'll probably just lower your monthly payment. Don't forget that how much a loan ultimately costs you is always a function of both the interest rate *and* the loan term. It's not unusual to get excited by a change in your monthly cash flow only to realize that you'll end up paying more over the life of the loan.

If the goal is to be aggressive in getting out of debt, you want to use debt reshuffling to make your payments *go further*, not to reduce them.

TAXES

BASIC TAX ASIDE

You don't pay your marginal tax rate on all of your income. You fill the brackets sequentially with rising income. When people get angry that some small amount of money "pushed them into a higher bracket," they are demonstrating a fundamental misunderstanding of the US tax code. Being in a higher bracket reduces the marginal value of the next dollar earned, but it doesn't retroactively reduce all of your earnings. What this does mean, however, is that the take-home value of each additional unit of your work does decrease in higher brackets. If moonlighting at $200/hour ended up being $122 instead of $150 after taxes, you might choose to work fewer extra night shifts in the ED.

STUDENT LOAN INTEREST TAX DEDUCTION

You may have heard that student loan payments are tax deductible. This is unfortunately only partially true: a relatively small portion of your student loan interest is deductible, at least probably while you're still a resident.

- Max $2,500 can be deducted per year

- Note that the student loan tax deduction is an "above the line deduction," meaning that you can take it even though you are likely not itemizing your deductions.

Remember the difference between a deduction and a credit. Deductions reduce your taxable income (thus saving you a percentage based on your marginal tax rate). Credits, on the other hand, are a dollar per dollar back.

A single resident making the typical resident salary without any additional income will generally qualify for the full $2,500 deduction.

That same resident will be in the 22% tax bracket, meaning that the deduction will save him less than one-fourth of that: $550. Better than a kick in the pants but nothing to get too excited about.

This is an example of how the government incentivizes certain behaviors through the tax code. For comparison, though it is a below the line deduction requiring itemization, you can generally deduct every penny of mortgage interest paid up to the house value of $1 million on your first and second homes. Despite what you hear from the politicians, perhaps the government prefers concrete foundations to educational ones.

For most residents with average loans, every dollar you spend on your loans during training will be dollars spent on interest because most residents face negative amortization during residency. If you consolidate your loans when you graduate, you will likely automatically max out the deduction the first year regardless of your actual monthly payments (i.e. even if you have $0 payments). This may seem counterintuitive, but the reason for this is that the IRS considers your new consolidation loan to "pay off" all of the uncapitalized interest that accrued while you were in school. Make sure to look at the 1098-E form your servicer sends you (and if they don't send it, you can usually download it from their website). You'll need it come tax time.

Every year thereafter you'll probably max it out with actual payments until you enter the phase-out.

Modified adjusted gross income (MAGI) limits (2018) for the student loan interest tax deduction:

- Full deduction: $65,000 if single, $135,000 if married

- Reduced by phase-out: $65k-$80k if single, $135k-165k if married

- Get nothing: >$80k if single, >$165k if married

Corollaries:

- The IDR payments for a resident will nearly always max out this deduction, no problem. Sadly, a significant portion of a resident's PAYE/REPAYE payments will be nondeductible, even more so for IBR.

- Borrowers in PAYE/REPAYE receiving the full $2,500 deduction will reduce monthly payments the following year by about $20.

- Attendings will generally get nothing. Residents in high cost of living areas may not either. Moonlighters ditto.

LIFETIME LEARNING CREDIT

- You can get a *credit* of up to $2,000 to cover tuition expenses. The details are readily available online and baked into TurboTax, but the credit amounts to 20% of the first $10,000 of tuition and fees for individuals making up to $65k and married couples up to $131k.

Most residents will get this credit when filing taxes during their intern spring for the fiscal year covering the second half of MS4 and first half of intern year, but if they had filed taxes every year of medical school (and aren't still a dependent on their parents return), they could have received this credit all four years. That's because according to the IRS:

Expenses qualify even if "paid with borrowed funds."

> *You can claim a lifetime learning credit for qualified education expenses paid with the proceeds of a loan. You use the expenses to figure the lifetime learning credit for the year in which the expenses are paid, not the year in which the loan is repaid. Treat loan disbursements sent directly to the educational institution as paid on the date the institution credits the student's account.*

So, don't forget to take this credit if you paid anything in taxes. Since the credit is per tax return based on "academic periods" (e.g. semesters) and not per calendar year, you can squeeze out 5 credits from the 4 years of medical school (spring MS1, spring MS2, spring MS3, spring MS4, spring Intern year). That's up to $10,000, if you would have ever owed that much to begin (it's a "non-refundable" credit, which means that it won't reduce your tax balance below zero).

RETIREMENT SAVINGS CONTRIBUTIONS CREDIT (SAVER'S CREDIT)

The Saver's Credit is an awesome credit that a lot of residents unfortunately won't qualify for. As an incentive for low-income workers to save for retirement, it has pretty strict income limits.

- Gives you a percentage back on retirement contributions up to $2,000 (a maximum of $1,000 back)

- Can't be student more than 5 months of the year (ruining this for interns)

CREDIT % PER AGI	MARRIED FILING JOINTLY	HEAD OF HOUSEHOLD	ALL OTHER FILERS
50% OF CONTRIBUTION	Up to $38,000	Up to $28,500	Up to $19,000
20% OF CONTRIBUTION	$38,001 - $41,000	$28,501 - $30,750	$19,001 - $20,500
10% OF CONTRIBUTION	$41,001 - $63,000	$30,751 - $47,250	$20,501 - $31,500
NO CREDIT	AGI > $63,000	AGI > $47,250	AGI > $31,500

The credit is good for a fraction of up to a $2,000 contribution to any retirement plan (403(b)/401(k)/Roth IRA/etc.), so for basically only for married residents without working spouses and even then at the 10% level (so $200). It's actually a $2k contribution per year per spouse, so it's really up to a free $400 ($200 x 2). Employer matches and pensions don't affect this, and it's a credit (not a deduction) so you get this money as cash.

The downside is that the only residents who will get this are those married with non-working spouses, and even then, residents in many locations and of increasing seniority will earn too much.

The plus side is that this can be a great deal for a low-earning spouse while you're in school, particularly if your spouse puts the money away in a Roth IRA. The free money can really reduce the pain of starting your plans for the future since the government is actually paying you to put money away (when you're broke).

The final downside is that this is also a "non-refundable" credit.

EARNED INCOME CREDIT

The Earned Income Tax Credit is a *refundable* tax credit available to "low to moderate" income folks. You get it just for earning some income (but not too much). Example AGI limits from 2018:

- $15,310 with no Qualifying Children ($21,000 if married filing jointly)

- $40,402 with one Qualifying Child ($46,102 if married filing jointly)

- $45,898 with two Qualifying Children ($51,598 if married filing jointly)

- $49,289 with three or more Qualifying Children ($54,998 if married filing jointly)

And investment income must also be less than $3,500 for the year.

For 2018, the maximum Earned Income Tax Credit per taxpayer was:

- $520 with no Qualifying Children

- $3,468 with one Qualifying Child

- $5,728 with two Qualifying Children

- $6,444 with three or more Qualifying Children

You must either have kids or be 25-years-old or older to get the credit, so if you have any income and this situation applies, make sure to file your taxes and get some free money. This is one of the only ways to get a real refund.

CONTRIBUTING TOWARD RETIREMENT

ABOUT RETIREMENT ACCOUNTS:

Note that when you place money into a pre-tax retirement account, you receive a tax *deferral* and not a true *deduction* or credit. You're deducting it from this year's taxes, but you're going to pay money on the distribution (when you take the money out) instead of the contribution (or in a Roth, on the contribution but not the distribution). Contrast that with the mortgage interest tax deduction, which is a true tax deduction: you simply get to keep the taxes that would be due on that money, period.

This isn't to say that the tax deferral doesn't have real tax benefits—it does! It's just that quantifying this benefit isn't as simple as taking the deduction and multiplying it by your marginal tax rate to get your savings. In a pretax account, you get to earn investment gains on money that *would* have been lost to taxes, even if the total income eventually gets taxed. Likewise, you won't pay taxes on any dividends or investment growth itself while the money remains in the account. Leave it alone and the number will generally get bigger and bigger over time. The exact retirement contribution tax benefits will depend on the tax bracket (federal + state) when you contribute, the tax bracket (federal + state) when you take a distribution, the earnings of the investment, and the length of time invested.

On a related note, it's actually good to have a combination of both pre- and after-tax retirement accounts such that you can combine withdrawals from them in retirement to limit taxes. Remember we talked about "filling up" tax brackets as you increase in income, so the idea is to use a combination: taxable pre-tax money until you fill up the cheap tax brackets and then switching to Roth money to avoid the increased marginal tax rates at higher income levels.

If your tax bracket at contribution and distribution are the same (both state and federal), the pretax and aftertax options are equivalent.

But most importantly, using these accounts works in your favor.

GET THE EMPLOYER-MATCH

Many employers offer a match on retirement contributions. These can take multiple forms: 100% match up to 3% of compensation, 50% match up to 5%, 100% match up to 4% vesting 20% every year of employment over 5 years, etc.

If your employer offers matching contributions, then you should contribute up to the match limit. Whatever system they use, it's free money. Obviously, if you're training in a high cost of living area and surviving on ramen you steal from a roommate you found on Craigslist, then I guess never mind.

From there, if you have more money, what to do next depends on the status of your loans and your risk tolerance.

IF YOU NEED TO PAY OFF YOUR LOANS:

There are no investments that are *guaranteed* to outperform the interest rate on your student loans, so in the event you plan on paying them off yourself (i.e. not going to stay in academics/public service and achieve PSLF), then you'll need to decide how risk tolerant you are: the certainty of paying down moderate-to-high interest debt versus the relative uncertainty of investing. If you're in REPAYE, as we discussed earlier, pretax retirement savings reduce your AGI, increase your subsidy, and decrease your effective interest rate. So that's one reason to invest.

For loans with interest rates in the 5-7% range, the math favors taking extra income and filling up your tax-advantaged accounts before putting extra money toward your loans. In the long term, this is likely to work out in your favor given historical investment returns. In the short term, market volatility can have impressive effects on investor psychology. If you choose to invest over paying off your loans, don't change plans when the market inevitably dips. In fact, when it dips is (perhaps counterintuitively) the best time to invest. One of the "perks" of retirement accounts is that you generally can't use the money without penalties, so it's difficult to sabotage yourself even if you get spooked. Do yourself a favor and invest in low-cost passive index funds and don't pay attention to what happens.

If you're leaning toward the predictability of repayment and are doing IDR making only partial interest payments, then you could put that money you wanted to use toward your loans temporarily in an interest-bearing savings account (e.g. Ally bank) or CD until you have enough money saved up to pay all the accrued interest so you can finally lower the principal and actually slow the rate of interest accrual. That way you can make a little bit of extra interest on the money earmarked for your loans before putting it to its intended use.

If your effective REPAYE rate is low or you've already refinanced to a lower interest rate, your money will go even farther in a retirement account than paying down low-interest loans, assuming you can take the financial uncertainty and loss of liquidity. If you can't, just pay off those loans and be content in watching the number drop.

IF YOU'RE HOPING FOR PSLF:

If you've already saved up a 2-3-month emergency fund and are making supplemental income you don't need but are attempting to qualify for PSLF, then you *really* don't want to pay down your loans directly. Any dollar you spend toward your loans is another that won't be forgiven by PSLF. If you're not sure but are in REPAYE making interest-only payments anyway, then again chipping away at your interest isn't going to make a big long-term dent since nothing is capitalizing anyway. We discussed this at length in the Maximizing PSLF chapter.

While Roth (after-tax) 401(k)s and 403(b)s are generally great options for low-earning residents, they have no effect on student loan payments. To reiterate: only contributing to a *pretax* account will reduce your adjusted gross income and lower your income-driven repayment. A $50,000-earning resident making a $2,500 403(b) contribution will reduce their total repayment the following year by $250 (an automatic 10% return). Ultimately, you may decide that the Roth version still makes sense, especially if you are concerned taxes will be higher when you retire decades from now.

Whichever you choose, you don't have to feel bad about choosing to invest in a tax-advantaged retirement account. The tax savings and likely yield of your investment may not always add up to more than the interest accruing on your loans at any given time, but it's still a financially responsible decision. Ultimately, if forgiveness is a possibility, it'll be safer to invest than throwing money into a loan that you might not need to pay off anyway.

MAXIMIZING YOUR TAX-ADVANTAGED SPACE:

First, max out your employer match. If you still have more money, the order of account filling again depends on whether or not you have loans and are trying to maximize the theoretical yield and flexibility of the retirement contribution or maximize PSLF. We're double-covering this information because it's important forever.

What percentage of your income you need to save for retirement depends on how much you make, how many years you'll be working, and how much you want to retire on. 15-20% of gross income is commonly recommended. Less than 10% is considered imprudent over the long term. You may not be able to do as much early in your career as you get settled, but the earlier you start the more time you give each dollar to grow.

THE ROTH IRA:

A great option for residents (especially non-PSLF bound) is to try to max out your Roth IRA up to the annual limit of $5,500 (and the same amount for your spouse for a total of $11,000, if the situation applies/allows). That's as much (and probably more) than you're likely to have sitting around as a resident. In this situation, you are putting after-tax money away while in a relatively low tax bracket that can then grow and be dispersed tax-free.

If your combined household income is above the Roth limit (single $120,000 phase-out/ineligible at $135,000; married $189,000 phase-out/ineligible at $199,000 in 2017), then you should consider the "backdoor Roth IRA," which is a Roth conversion that involves moving money originally contributed to a traditional IRA over to a Roth account. (You'll want to Google it if this applies to you.)

IF YOUR ROTH IRA IS FULL:

Consider utilizing a Health Savings Account if available, as we discussed in the Maximizing PSLF chapter. HSAs are so-called "stealth IRAs" that allow you to put money away triple-tax-free (no taxes on the contribution, earnings, or distribution) for health expenditures or like a regular 401(k) for non-health expenditures. HSAs are offered in association with High Deductible Health Plans, so these aren't universally available. Don't confuse them with the much more common Flexible Spending Accounts (FSA), which do allow for tax-free contributions for health care expenditures but also must be used up annually or the money is forfeited.

Then you'd likely want to sock away the money in either your employer 401(k)/403(b) (if they provide one) or a solo 401(k) (that you can set up if you moonlight and receive income as an independent contractor on a 1099). If you become a loan-free resident, you'd likely benefit from the Roth option of those accounts if one is available. If not, a regular pretax retirement account will work just fine.

IF YOU CAN SAVE MORE THAN THAT:

In order to need even more tax-efficient saving options, you'll have managed to max out a Roth IRA for yourself (and your spouse) and max out the personal contribution limit of your 401(k)/403(b)

($19,000 in 2019) (and your spouse too if they have enough income to do the same). That's considerably more than most residents can afford and as much (and often more) than a lot of early career docs can swing.

Your next options are a 457(b) account (another pretax retirement vehicle commonly offered at academic institutions with another $19k per year limit) or a solo/individual 401(k) (as mentioned above), which is an individual account you can start as the sole proprietor of your one-(wo)man 1099-earning business. While the $189 personal limit is summed across all accounts, your "business" can put up to 20% of its profits to your 401(k) on your behalf (25% if you structure your business as a corporation) up to the annual (2017) contribution limit of $56,000 total (personal + profit-sharing).

So, for example, if you had maxed out your $19k contribution to your hospital 403(b) and then you made another $10k moonlighting as an independent contractor, you could basically put another $2,000 into the individual 401(k). Note: the calculation of acceptable contributions for a solo 401(k) is a bit more complicated than multiplying by 0.2, but online calculators exist, and tax software can also do this for you. There are a bunch of options for opening a Solo 401(k) account, including companies that allow for both Roth and traditional pre-tax options, so you can choose how much tax you feel like paying now versus later.

If you have kids, and everything else is maxed, you could start a 529 account to start paying for college. Your state may offer you a deduction for the 529 contribution, but the feds do not. In general, you want to have your own financial house in order before trying to pay for your kid's college.

WHAT ABOUT MY MORTGAGE?

If you own a house or condo and thus have a mortgage, paying it down faster makes less sense financially than contributing to tax-advantaged retirement accounts given the currently available interest rates, with the main practical exceptions that, psychologically, having no mortgage makes people happy, and you can also potentially get the money back earlier in your lifetime if you need to by selling the house or refinancing.

Unlike every other loan you have, mortgage interest payments are generally completely tax deductible, which means that your effective rate is even lower than what it is on paper. Paying down the mortgage is generally a better option once retirement accounts are maxed.

ROTH CONVERSIONS DURING SCHOOL OR RESIDENCY

If you have any pretax retirement accounts from a former employer, a Roth conversion during school or even residency is something to consider. This means taking your previously untaxed contributions and converting them to an after-tax Roth account by paying the income tax on them now.

Doing this as a student with little or no income can result in no taxes due on the converted money, which can then be withdrawn tax-free in retirement. Clever conversion timing can sometimes shield income from the taxman entirely.

CLOSING THOUGHTS

Ultimately, even as a resident, you're already starting the retirement game late compared to those who entered the job market directly without an expensive 4-year graduate degree. The more years your money is sitting in an account, the more years it has a chance to grow. But more than that, even putting away a small amount of money (which is unlikely to make a significant difference in your overall portfolio) jumpstarts the savings behavior early. And *that* will keep you honest so that you can "pay yourself first" when you really begin to make the money that will be very tempting to spend and lose to lifestyle inflation.

There are no "wrong" or "bad" choices between saving for retirement and paying off your loans responsibly because both are "good" things to do with your money. Everyone has different financial goals and risk tolerance. In doing either you'll do much better than the average person.

Do yourself a favor and at least contribute to the company match during training (if one is available). Make contributing to your retirement something automatic: a payroll deduction that you never really see, so that you're doing right by yourself from the very start of your career.

THE FUTURE

Prognostication is a uniquely human trait that, at least when it comes to matters of money, we fail at as a species. You can't time the market, professional investors can't beat the index over the long term, and no one can predict interest rate changes. The same could easily be said for forecasting changes to student loan terms and re-payment programs.

THE FUTURE OF PSLF

The multimillion-dollar question is the fate of PSLF. The project-ed costs and utilization of this program are far beyond the initial estimates, and it seems self-evident that both lawmakers and the public will not enjoy the coming news barrage of millionaire neuro-surgeons getting their debt wiped away while driving BMWs. Even with a growing desire (on the Democratic side) to make college free, that doesn't mean the current iteration of unlimited non-means-tested forgiveness is likely to last forever.

On the other hand, even when/if PSLF changes or is canceled in the future, the current PSLF program is baked into the language of the master promissory note you signed when you took out your loans.

Other than simply defunding the program and dealing with the in-evitable lawsuits, it's hard to see how the feds could legally ruin the program for old borrowers.

If you are curious, you can read a complete Direct loan master prom-issory note here: https://studentloans.gov/myDirectLoan/download-PDF.action?fileName=SUBUNSUBMPN (if that link doesn't work, just Google "master promissory note" and you'll come across the government's official example). Despite being a binding legal doc-ument, it's written in mostly plain English.

For *future* borrowers, there are essentially four options:

- The program might be canceled entirely

- The forgiven amount might be capped (perhaps $57.5k)

- A "means test" might be instituted such that high-income individuals will not have their loans forgiven.

- REPAYE-type loophole closures (e.g. removing the payment cap and MFS-loophole) are applied to PAYE and IBR for new borrowers, thus ensuring that high-income years reduce the total amount of forgiveness.

Capping forgiveness was the proposal of the outgoing Obama administration. Trump, as we'll discuss below, has favored option 1.

THE 2017 BUDGET PROPOSAL

This is the future that never was. The Obama administration's 2017 budget proposal (again) proposed capping PSLF at $57,500 (the borrowing limit for undergraduates) to "protect against institutional practices that may further increase student indebtedness, while ensuring the program provides generous relief for students committed to public service." A capped PSLF would change the calculus for most physicians. Certainly, those entering academia would enjoy the free money, but PSLF would lose its panacea-like status as a way to ignore the absurdly high cost of becoming a physician.

The proposal also recommended a single one-size fits all PAYE for new borrowers in 2017 that would also remove the payment cap (like REPAYE), ensuring that "high-income, high-balance borrowers to pay an equitable share of their earnings as their incomes rise." That's us, by the way.

They also recommended closing the married filing separately loophole in this new plan.

In the proposal, Perkins would become a DIRECT loan (and thus automatically eligible for IDR and PSLF), which is good, but then become unsubsidized (which is bad). In the end, the Perkins program was simply shuttered.

Overall, these recommendations were essentially just parting thoughts of an administration on its way out, particularly as the Democrats lost the presidency. If Clinton had won, then these proposals would likely illustrate the overall trend of things to come. But even then, I want to point out that the floated ideas never involved anyone who had already borrowed and made financial decisions and plans:

> *However, students who borrowed their first loans prior to July 1, 2017, would continue to be able to select among the existing repayment plans for loans borrowed to fund their current course of study.*

If you'd already signed a promissory note, you would've received the old rules.

THE WARREN ULTIMATUM

Before she and many democratic candidates started proposing free college, there had already been proposed legislation from Elizabeth Warren to allow loan holders to refinance their loans internally within the federal system to the new rates currently offered to current borrowers. A medical student graduating in 2012, for example, carries loans predominately at 6.8%. However new unsubsidized graduate loan rates are currently 6%. More recently, Warren and friends proposed the "Student Loan Tax Relief Act," which would make all loan forgiveness under any program (i.e. IDR) tax-free.

Unfortunately, this hasn't happened and, unless Democrats gain a majority in the Senate during the 2020 elections, anything like it is highly unlikely to happen in the near future. While it would be nice, it would be imprudent to consider this remote possibility when you make your plans.

THE TRUMP PLAN

Candidate Trump unveiled his vision for student loans as a single choice IDR plan at 12.5% of AGI (essentially splitting the difference between PAYE and IBR) with all undergraduate loans forgiven after 15 years and graduate loans forgiven after 30 years. The PSLF program would be canceled.

Ironically, despite the discussion of the doctor's loophole within public service loan forgiveness, Trump's original plan would actually have resulted in even more "rich" private practice docs having their loans forgiven in large amounts. Likewise, imagine how much easier it would be to have your loans forgiven while working part time or while saving for retirement. Part-time work is not eligible for PSLF, but with your reduced income, your monthly payments toward the 15-year universal forgiveness would've been low. Tack on as much pretax retirement saving as you can manage and voila, even better. The Congressional budget office did weigh in and unsurprisingly determined that this plan was costly and terrible. While undoubtedly true for the nation, it may have been nice for some physicians.

President Trump's actual 2018 and 2019 budget proposals kept Candidate Trump's plan for undergraduates but extended the forgiveness timeline to 30 years for graduate students. PSLF would be abolished alongside all currently offered IDR plans.

Why this? Because Trump's stated goal is to get the government away from its large role in supplying and managing student loan debt, of which Americans already hold more than 1.4 trillion dollars. Certainly stretching the forgiveness timeline for graduate debt to 30 years would make private refinancing a better deal, which one imagines is partly the point. Betsy DeVos, Trump's completely unqualified pick for Education Secretary, has spent her entire tenure trying to limit student loan consumer protections in order to protect business profits and ostensibly limit government spending, so it would seem nothing good would ever come down the pipeline during this administration.

That said, this proposal is being ignored. Presidents make "budget proposals," but Congress makes budgets. Obama's request for a much less seismic PSLF-cap went ignored for two years in a row despite Republican majorities in both the House and the Senate, and student loans remain a hot-button topic. Trump's initial proposal was similarly ignored last year for the 2018 budget, and it returned without major change for the 2019 proposal.

If implemented, Trump's administration has already specifically stated that the new single plan option would only be mandatory for new borrowers (those with their earliest loans in 2019). Current borrowers who have already signed their promissory notes under the old regime will be able to continue in the current convoluted scheme. Whether or not older borrowers would be eligible for the new plan or not could go either way, but the recent trend has been toward broad availability and simplification (so probably yes, but why would you want to?).

Republicans in congress, for their part, unveiled their dream/plan in late 2017 for borrowers to pay 15% of their discretionary incomes toward student debt with no option for forgiveness. Instead, borrowers would make payments until they finally paid the amount due under a 10-year repayment plan (including interest). Now *that* would be a kick in the gut for a lot of borrowers, some of whom would likely be making student loan payments with their social security benefits!

While the Trump plan still does not address the cost of education, the Republican House plan would likely do more to combat cost inflation. Under this proposal, everyone pays for his/her education no matter how long it takes (presumably unless you die first). For people considering the value of another degree, the Republican tax cuts are a drop in the bucket if your wages will be garnished for your entire career because you never make enough to actually pay off your loans.

But for you, the current borrower, it's important to keep in mind that the MPN is a legal contract. That contract currently includes PSLF, REPAYE, PAYE, IBR, and ICR as options. So, there's a reason why grandfathering changes is the standard practice; it's not just beneficence.

Fearmongers about changes to government repayment programs and forgiveness options usually have a vested interest in these changes, because any decrease in the quality of government programs or forgiveness will push people into the arms of private refinancing companies, from which they earn commissions. **There is no evidence or precedent that any future changes will affect existing borrowers.**

FINAL THOUGHTS ON THE FUTURE

There is no doubt that the Congressional budget office grossly underestimated the cost of the public service loan forgiveness program. For one, they apparently had no idea how good of a deal it would be for many large volume graduate student borrowers. They also didn't anticipate how the availability of large-volume forgiveness would essentially subsidize egregious tuition increases, not limited to but especially among private and for-profit law and medical schools, which often tout loan forgiveness as a hand-wavy means of writing off absurdly expensive costs of attendance. PSLF is here for now, but it's definitely a target.

Despite the doom and gloom, the fact that congress recently temporarily *expanded* the program via the Temporary Expanded Public Service Loan Forgiveness (TEPSLF) would suggest that the end isn't as close as some had feared.

Nevertheless, there are an increasing number of schools charging tuitions that would be financially catastrophic for those entering many specialties in the absence of loan forgiveness programs. For the unfortunate students of these institutions, the baked-in forgiveness of PAYE or REPAYE may ultimately be a viable choice, but it is undesirable for most borrowers to be on the hook for 20-25 years of payments (likely the bulk of their career) followed by a large lump sum due in taxes (even if this would please and profit the government).

The future is rapidly coming where becoming a doctor in many fields will be a financially unsound choice.

THE WORKFLOW

A lot of this book has been detailed background coupled with an in-depth discussion of your options and considerations for evaluating student loan debt and picking a repayment strategy. Admittedly, some of the details and scenarios we've discussed do not pertain to many borrowers, but the goal here isn't to tell you what to do so much as give you the tools you need to make your own strong informed decision.

Here's the brief version to summarize the simple approach, both as a conclusion and for those of you who stopped caring at page 7:

STEP 1:

Try not to borrow so much money.

STEP 2:

Consolidate your federal loans into a Direct Consolidation after graduation and before starting internship.

STEP 3:

Pick your (first) repayment plan, probably REPAYE, maybe PAYE, hopefully not IBR.

For most folks:

Single: REPAYE

Married with non-working spouse: REPAYE

Married with working spouse: Compare REPAYE and PAYE.

- If you get a subsidy with REPAYE, then REPAYE. If you don't, then PAYE.

- If attempting PSLF, then compare PAYE payments with filing taxes jointly and separately. If MFS saves you more money than you lose in extra taxes, then probably PAYE with consideration of filing taxes separately.

- If definitely not doing PSLF, consider private refinance, but probably still end up waiting until after training. Always compare private rates with the REPAYE *effective* rate.

Step 3.1:

Don't spend too much money.

Step 3.2:

Seriously.

Step 3.3:

If relevant, maximize REPAYE and PSLF benefits by minimizing your adjusted gross income through retirement accounts and other "income-reducing" measures.

Step 3.4:

If you're not sure about PSLF, consider putting extra money toward retirement or in something safe like an interest-bearing online savings account as a "loan payoff slush fund" that can be deployed if your plans change.

STEP 4:

Stay on top of annual IDR income certifications. If considering PSLF, file employment certification forms annually as well.

STEP 5:

Keep abreast of coming changes to your finances, career, and family to adjust your plan accordingly.

- If you originally choose REPAYE and are on the cusp of personal or spousal income increases, weigh the possibility of switching to PAYE if you'll be losing your PAYE eligibility (partial financial hardship) or breaking past the standard payment-cap.

- Likewise, consider filing taxes separately in PAYE/IBR.

STEP 6:

Eventually get rid of those student loans, either via PSLF or paying it off as fast as you can.

If you're an attending not bound for PSLF and you're able to make progress paying down your loans, then you likely make too much money to have any benefit from federal loans and should consider refinancing.

When it comes to actually paying off a loan, a lower rate is a lower rate, and a shorter term always reduces interest costs.

CALCULATORS

I've put this brief section at the end because I believe it's important to understand how the loans and repayment options work before plugging and chugging. It's very easy to use a calculator to get an incorrect answer if you ask it the wrong question.

Most calculators will give you a "first month" payment based on your actual inputs and an estimated "final month" payment and total repayment/forgiveness numbers based on multiple assumptions. The first month payment is gold. The final one is only good for illustrative purposes at best (and usually useless).

You'll generally be better off calculating a new "first month" payment for each year of your repayment and iterating over years (which you can do all at once with the Doctored Money and Student Loan Planner calculators below) than to use any calculator's predictions if any of your choices seem close.

THE FEDERAL STUDENT AID REPAYMENT ESTIMATOR

The original. You can put in your loans, your spouse's loans, family size and residence, your income, and your spouse's income and it will spit out your monthly payments and estimated repayment for every federal repayment plan in a single comparison table. Very handy. It can pull in your loans if you log in to your FSA account. Otherwise it will take you a minute to put all the info (you'll be faster if you just input a single "virtual consolidation" if you haven't consolidated), but you can then quickly see how income changes monthly payment as well as the difference in tax filing status.

Link: https://studentloans.gov/myDirectLoan/repaymentEstimator.action

DOCTORED MONEY

A detailed online embedded spreadsheet. Sometimes runs a bit slowly, but it allows you to plot out and compare all of your federal repayment plan options over a 10-year span. Well-designed with a bunch of nice tables and graphical depictions, including your annual REPAYE subsidy and effective REPAYE interest rate. It's perfect for figuring out if PSLF is for you. If needed, you'll have to compare any potential private refinance separately.

Link: https://www.doctoredmoney.org/student-debt/loan-repayment-calculator

STUDENT LOAN HERO

Multiple single purpose calculators. Useful to quickly determine first month payments, as well as the costs of deferment/forbearance, your weighted loan interest rate, comparing refinancing term lengths.

Link: https://studentloanhero.com/calculators/

STUDENT LOAN PLANNER

Detailed Excel spreadsheet. Like the Doctored Loans calculator with the addition and heavy branding of private financing. A little intimidating to use at first, but if you put a few minutes in, it'll also give you detailed results in one place.

Link: https://www.studentloanplanner.com/free-student-loan-calculator/ (requires submitting your email)

FINANCIAL ROUNDS

This is a relatively new project from a CFP and includes another PSLF calculator so that you can check your work.

Link: https://www.financialrounds.com/tools/pslf-calculator/

MEDLOANS

Like the federal loan estimator but also includes PSLF estimates. It can also import your loans from NSLDS, which is neat.

Link: https://apps.aamc.org/first-gloc-web/ (requires AAMC login)

HELPFUL FURTHER READING

INCOME-DRIVEN REPAYMENT PLANS

The basics, with helpful tables and links

Link: https://studentaid.ed.gov/sa/repay-loans/understand/plans/income-driven

INCOME-DRIVEN REPAYMENT Q & A

26 pages of official government answers to very important questions, written in plain English.

Link: https://studentaid.ed.gov/sa/sites/default/files/income-driven-repayment-q-and-a.pdf

AAMC EDUCATION DEBT MANAGER

The newly updated 2017 version is a pretty slick and nicely-present-ed comprehensive review of the basics if you didn't like the way they were described here. Free and worth a read but missing some of the nuances.

Link: https://members.aamc.org/eweb/upload/Education%20 Debt%20Manager%20for%20Graduating%20Medical%20 School%20Students--2017.pdf

DOCTORED MONEY

Nice, new, and growing non-profit site with excellent discussions of federal repayment options. I particularly like their new loan scenarios page.

Link: https://www.doctoredmoney.org/ (https://www.doctoredmon-ey.org/loan-scenarios)

GOOD LUCK

After a few hours of counting cents and trying to make sense of your options, it's worth noting that real life can easily get in the way of almost every repayment strategy. You could get married and your spouse could have a ton of student loans, making REPAYE or even federal forgiveness programs make sense when they didn't before. Or, you could get married and your high-earning spouse could have no student loans, completely changing the effectiveness of the RE-PAYE program. You could enter academia by accident. You could end up finding a private practice job that you can't pass up. You may decide to work part-time to care for your family in one way or another and thus no longer qualify for PSLF even if you do work in academia. You might quit medicine altogether to pursue your dream of making bespoke soap.

Unless you only have a small amount of loans and paying them down as fast as possible is the obvious solution, anything else you do may require revision over time. This is particularly true if the calculus between options such as paying your loans off and trying to get them forgiven doesn't differ by large amounts and depends on the relative details of monthly payments and shifting interest rates. The beauty of this situation is that as long as you're proactive, you'll be fine. While the initial return on your investment in medicine is terrible, it generally works out in your favor over a 30-year career.

You should run your current and possible numbers into one of the various free calculators online to help you make decisions, but you should be wary of accepting any long-term predictions. The problem is that it's hard for any calculator to demonstrate your options accurately as a proactive young physician. The fact that you've read this book or want to use a calculator at all means that the simple assumptions these usually make don't apply. But taking the time to input different scenarios into a calculator and plotting out your strategy *does* work.

As we've discussed, people trying to aggressively repay their loans who choose an income-driven repayment plan like REPAYE during residency may be best served by refinancing privately to a short-term loan and even making extra payments as much as possible after completing training. But even this simple common scenario is difficult to capture in any available calculator.

You can test the assumptions yourself. You don't need to pay anyone anything, and if you did, the future could still invalidate your best-laid plans. Don't be a passive participant in your financial life. You've probably lived for years at 5, 6, or 7%, but now it's time to make change.

FEEDBACK?

I'd love to receive your feedback. This book is a living document and will benefit from your thoughts and experiences—just email me at ben@benwhite.com.

I'd also be grateful if you took the time to share what you've learned with others. We're all in this together.

Made in the USA
San Bernardino, CA
10 February 2020